WONDERS OF RADIOLOGY

Z.V. MAIZLIN

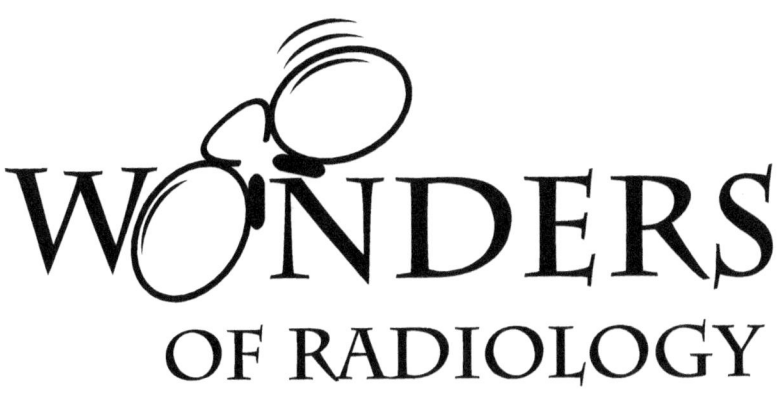

WONDERS

OF RADIOLOGY

NOT ONLY
FOR WONDERING
RADIOLOGISTS

ZEEV V. MAIZLIN, MD
Associate Professor
Department of Radiology
McMaster University
Hamilton, Ontario, Canada

TO THE MEMORY
OF MY FATHER
DR. SAMUEL N. MAIZLIN

Acknowledgements

The author expresses gratitude and appreciation to Ms Monika Ferrier, BA. Her dedication, creativeness, fluency in languages and ability to find the hidden helped to enrich this book with details and portraits. Highly qualified librarian, very knowledgeable and helpful, she supplied answers to many of my questions and never failed to fulfill any request.

My special thanks to my family, whose support and help made this book possible.

CONTENTS

PREFACE

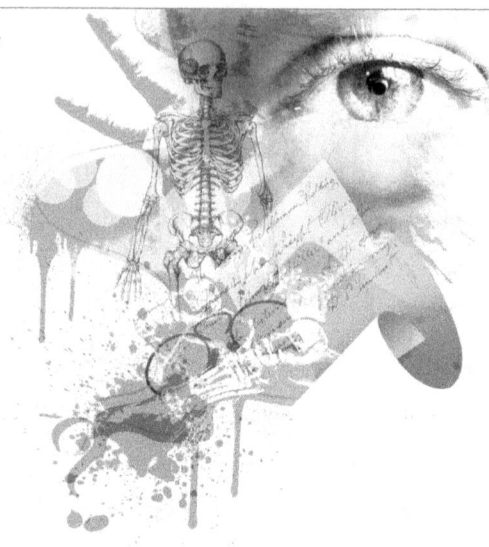

The Time When the World Was Held by Titans

The Seven Wonders of the Ancient World were the most remarkable man-made creations of classical antiquity. Radiology is young. It is barely 100 years old. How could this specialty be so developed to produce wonders of its own? 100 years ago the world lived in an incredible time when dreams and fantasy materialized in new inventions which changed daily life making it unrecognizable. This was the era when the first cars appeared on the roads. First planes flew in the sky. First submarines took people to the depths of the sea. The existence of new rays, unknown and mysterious, was announced. So mysterious, that their discoverer called them 'X'-rays using the mathematical designation for 'unknown'!

From the first days when the medical usefulness of new rays became apparent, physicians were thrilled and attracted to working with them. Never mind that the hazardous effects of their usage were poorly understood! X-rays could speed-up a career with promotion unheard of in the strict structure of already well-established medical specialties. Dealing with x-rays carried a potential of new research and publications. The rays were mysterious and attractive for the physicians and patients alike. They also could be a profitable business venture. People were ready to pay and rays' business potential was enormous.

Radiology could become for physicians what the railway was for the investors and industry in the mid 19th century and what Hi-Tech, computers and internet were in the late 20th century. Radiology was new and revolutionary. It held the promise of unlimited potential in diagnosis and treatment. Medical degree, openness to new technology, basic knowledge of work with electrical and photographic equipment – and other great perspectives were opening! To hang the tube on a photographic tripod! Manually operate the dynamo to produce the electrical current! With this equipment and lots of enthusiasm – the horizon was the limit!

Like during the gold rush, when people raced each other in common pursuit of new and highly lucrative goldfields, mystery, rivalry and even crime were involved in radiology history. The physician could bargain the award of a highly honored title for permission to import an X-ray machine. The radiologist, opening a highly successful roentgen laboratory, just barely escaped the attempt launched by the rival to get him out of the way with the chain of mysterious events that followed.

The greatest wonder of radiology is people. Those who developed it and made it the most advanced field of modern medicine. Many works have been published describing the initial steps and history of development of radiology in different countries. However, the contribution of some physicians to radiology crossed national borders. Names "engraved" in radiological signs became eponyms and are used now on all the continents and countries of the world. The usage of these names unites radiologists in Europe and Asia, America and Australia. Isn't it wonderful? But who were these people? Some of them were famous. International societies and awards were named after them. Names of others are almost lost in obscurity. No biographical details, no photographs! Nothing except the sign carrying the name!

Collection of the biographical details about these people took us on a search in immigration archives, old newspapers, telephone books of remote cities. It made us look for contact with family friends and descendants of these people. Years of seemingly fruitless attempts were disappointing. And at the moments of deepest desperation it came! The replies from the archives or libraries sparkled like the tiny glitter of precious stones. Pieces of information were assembled. Previously unpublished data and photographs were found! Sometimes hair stood on end when fascinating and interesting facts were uncovered while collecting material for this book. And what a wonderful light they shed on the history of radiology! These successes made a fascinating tour to the past exciting and fruitful.

We discovered that eponyms sometimes emerged as a result of a single article, which was not necessarily a significant step in the author's career. Quite frequently, people whose names are used now as eponyms of radiological signs, are actually known for their activity in other fields. Codman was a famous surgeon, Fraenkel was the famous pathologist and bacteriologist, Park – a pediatrician, Stierlin worked in fields of psychiatry and surgery.

An eponym in medicine is the name of a disease or a structure, based on or derived from the name of a person. Eponyms not only honor those who have valuably contributed to medicine. Eponyms play an important role in proper reporting and communication providing an efficient, easy and short way of describing signs and syndromes. Chronologically, most eponyms used in radiology today were created in the first half of the 20th century. No eponyms seem to be originating from articles published starting from the late 1970s. Some of them are still in active use, others, likely mirroring the progress of imaging and diagnostic techniques, are almost forgotten. An enormous number of medical articles are published. What transformed the description given in the article into the eponym? What gave life to the eponym? What defined how long and how renowned this "life" would be? Why did some eponyms become widely known and used in publications and in clinical practice while others are abandoned? Quite frequently, just a few sentences in the original article were picked up and cited creating the eponym. This initial citation, in fact, was the birth act for the eponym.

It is not easy to understand and define the process of the creation of eponyms. It seems that the personality, scientific and administrative status of the author did not play any role. Some of these people were rewarded and famous. Others were virtually unknown with just a few published works or even only one. Some of them worked in world known centers and some in middle size hospitals or private clinics.

This book provides an insight into the life and work of people who gave their name to the eponyms. These people belonged to the generation of Titans. Like Titans, they marked an early golden age of the new science, developed and shaped radiology, transforming it into an advanced, interesting and descriptive science.

Z.Maizlin
Lake Muskoka, Ontario, 2009

Heinrich Ernst Albers-Schönberg

Prometheus of the New Rays
Fame and Tragedy
The First Full Professor Of Radiology
The First Victim

Osteopetrosis or marble bone disease is an increased radiological density of the bones. It was described by Heinrich Ernst Albers-Schönberg in 1904, less than nine years after Roentgen's discovery of x-rays.

Heinrich Ernst Albers-Schönberg was born on January 21, 1865 in Hamburg. He came from the family of the royal merchants. His father, August Heinrich Schönberg, was adopted by the Albers family in Hamburg, and converted his name to Albers-Schönberg.

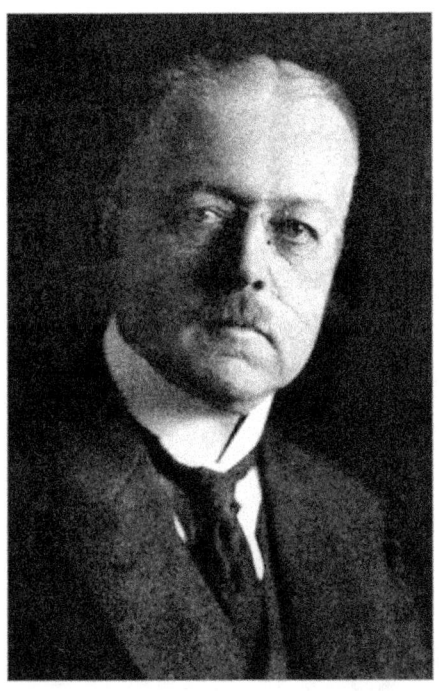

‖ *Heinrich Ernst Albers-Schönberg* *

With interruptions for the military service, Heinrich studied medicine in Tübingen and Leipzig, graduating in 1891. After working at the Leipzig Frauenklinik (Women's Hospital) of Dr. Zweifel he returned to his native Hamburg. He started his career in 1892 as an assistant physician in the department for women and children at the newly established Allgemeines Krankenhaus Hamburg-Eppendorf. For his self-sacrificing activity during the cholera epidemic, he was granted an education journey to Berlin and Vienna. In 1895 he settled as a practitioner

* *See Photographic Credits - p. 166*

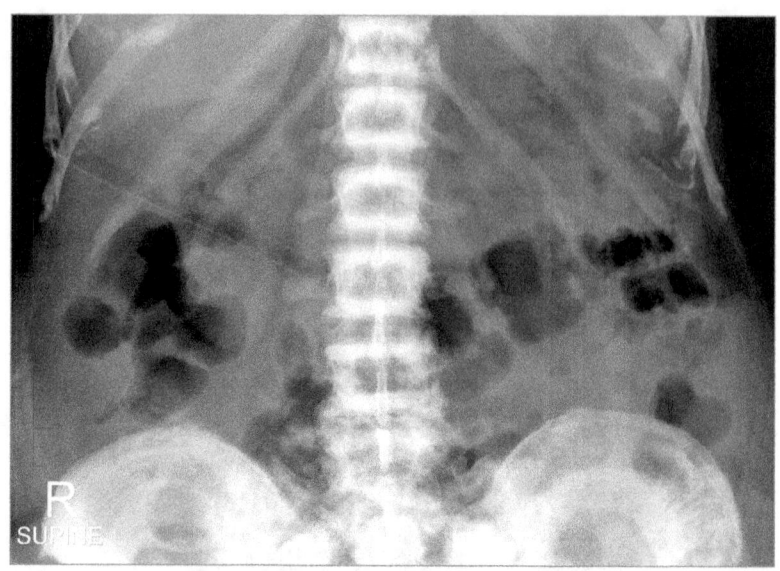

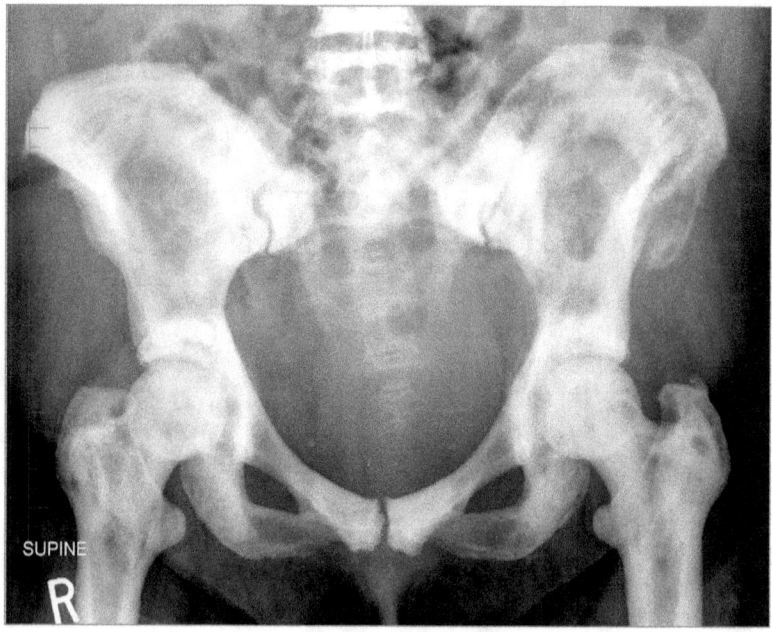

Osteopetrosis or marble bone disease.
Rugger jersey spine and increased density
of the pelvic bones.

in Hamburg. Tall, elegant, distinguished-looking, a Doctor of Medicine with glasses and a jauntily twirled mustache, he quickly became part of Hamburg society. He met Margaret, a young widow who came from the family of Senator Schroeder. They married and moved into a prestigious house on Hochallee 48. Soon Heinrich Albers-Schönberg became one among prosperous Hamburg doctors. He planned to devote himself to the treatment of female diseases.

However, the events which took place in November 1895 in the small city of Würzburg, 500 kilometers from Hamburg, changed the life of the young gynecologist. These events made him internationally famous, respected and prosperous. They took him to enormous sufferings and pain. His life never again was what it had been before. Meteoric rise and despair of cruel disease turned Heinrich Albers-Schönberg into Prometheus of the new rays and of medical research with his fame and great tragedy.

The discovery of Wilhelm Conrad Röntgen, 54-year old professor of physics from Würzburg, immediately became the sensation in Hamburg. Albers-Schönberg was fascinated reading Röntgen's brochure. He studied the report on the meeting of the Physikalisch-Medizinische Gesellschaft (Physical-Medical Society) of Würzburg from 23 January 1896. He could not stop looking at the first published x-ray.

Albers-Schönberg was always interested in

technology. He also was an avid amateur photographer. His still not so busy doctor's practice provided him with enough time for his hobbies. So in the next few months he became a frequent guest of Dr. Bernhard Walter in the Physikalische Staatsinstitut who had built an x-ray machine and started experiments with the new rays. Unfortunately, experiments could not last long. The tube became too hot. Walter invented water cooling for the tube which could now provide the beam of rays indefinitely. Now it was ready to be used in medicine!

On 20 March 1896, just two months after Röntgen's presentation, the first x-ray machine was put into service in the surgical department of Eppendorf Hospital. The tube for this machine was blown by glass-blower Becker in the small light bulb factory on the ground floor of the house at Bremer Reihe 14, which

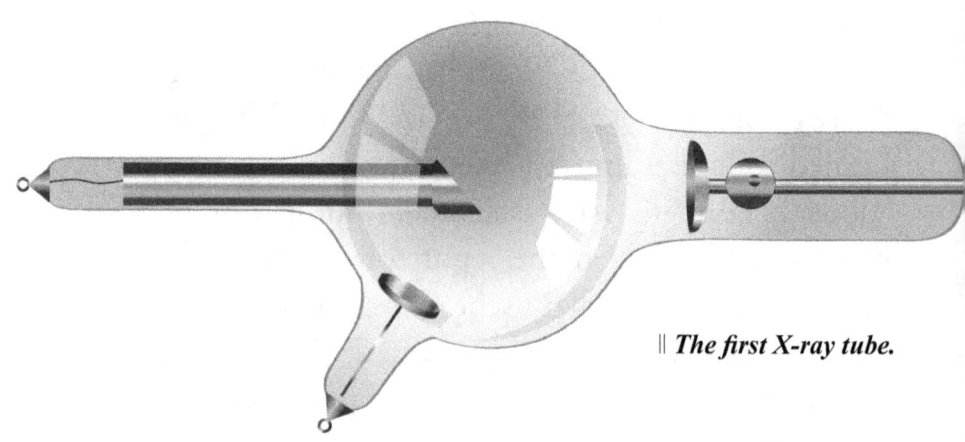

|| *The first X-ray tube.*

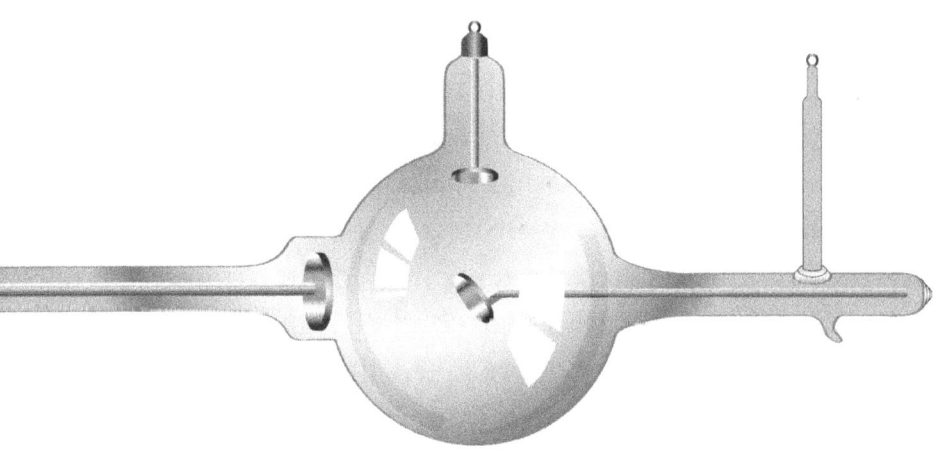

belonged to Carl Heinrich Florenz Müller. Albers-Schönberg visited the master Müller. He asked for the tube for the private radiology department which at that time existed only in his mind. Müller also was working on development of water-cooled anodes for X-ray tubes. Who could imagine in those days, full of enthusiasm and excitement, that x-ray would bring to the small factory of Florenz Müller, founded in 1865, great business success, transforming it to the international Hamburg company of C.H.F. Müller Röntgenwerk (Röntgenmüller). Master Florenz Müller was later awarded the Gold medal by the Roentgen Society of London for his improved water-cooled x-ray tubes. Suffering from complications of radiation damage he died in 1912. Fifteen years later his company was bought by Phillips giving birth to the future giant of the roentgen equipment.

A year after his first visit to Müller, in 1897

Albers-Schönberg, together with his colleague, Dr. Georg Deycke, established at Klopstockstraße 10 a private institution for the application of radiographic techniques to internal medicine. It was one of the first medical x-ray institutes in the world. Albers-Schönberg's stepson remembered the atmosphere of the x-ray cabinet: "For us children it always was terribly exciting when we were taken into the institute. The room was full of wires, cables and mysterious-looking instruments. Under the x-ray tubes father sometimes x-rayed our hands."

Albers-Schönberg gave up his gynecologic practice and concentrated his efforts entirely on radiology, becoming the first specialist in this field of medicine.

Albers-Schönberg had only occasional contact with Röntgen himself. He seldom corresponded with him and only later did they meet at the congress of the German Radiology Society. The reason for that was that Röntgen, a physicist and theorist, was hardly interested in the practical application of his rays. It was Albers-Schönberg's successor, Hermann Holthusen, who was the only doctor in the world who could say: "I have x-rayed Röntgen." In 1919, coming to Heidelberg for treatment, Röntgen confessed: "I've never seen an x-ray cabinet from the inside."

Although Röntgen cared little about the medical value of his rays, enthusiastic young doctors in Hamburg soon rallied around Albers-

Schönberg. In order to share and exchange rapidly collecting experience and scientific results, already in 1897 Albers-Schönberg and Deycke founded the radiology journal *Fortschritte auf dem Gebiete der Röntgenstrahlen*. Deycke's decision to leave for Constantinople (Istanbul of our days) was a blow for Albers-Schönberg. He tried to convince his friend to stay (the career run would then take Deycke to the climax of success, though far away from radiology, but would end with the infamous trial of 1931, the accusation and guilt of having caused the death of 77 Lübeck children, and his own death in obscurity with a broken heart). After Deycke's departure, Albers-Schönberg had to run the institute and the journal alone.

Doctors referred patients to Albers-Schönberg and Deycke where these patients had to be x-rayed and diagnosed. Before acquisition of each image, Albers-Schönberg examined the quality of the beam. There was then no measurement equipment and Albers-Schönberg based the process on testing the image of his own hand to check whether the rays were 'hard' or 'soft'. He had no idea that he was turning himself into the first victim of the new science. Since the moment he saw the image of an x-rayed hand he decided to use the x-rays for patients.

Who could imagine that the image of his own hand would become for him the harbinger of death!

Only a few months after opening his practice, Albers-Schönberg's hands were red. They ached at the slightest touch. In order not to have to show his inflamed hands, during work and in society he slipped on white silk gloves. In this manner, he could hide the signs of disaster. But he could not escape his destiny.

In those early days of radiology nobody knew to warn about the dangers of radiation. Being careless and unprotected, Albers-Schönberg developed radiation-induced neoplasia in his hands, thorax and shoulder, and in 1908, his right middle finger and left arm were amputated. He suffered from great pain in the last period of his life.

In 1903 he found a damaging effect of radiation on the reproductive glands of rabbits, a discovery which induced the development of effective methods of protection and research of sterilization.

In 1903 Albers-Schönberg was appointed radiologist to the Hamburg Hospital and two years later became head of radiology. In 1915 he moved to a similar post at Allgemeines Krankenhaus St. Georg, Hamburg. He had considerable talent for organization and design of a new radiographic department.

In 1904 Albers-Schönberg received the Grand Prize of the World Fair in St. Louis. His diagnostic x-ray pictures were far better in clarity than any of the competitors' work.

During World War I, Albers-Schönberg was awarded a Red Cross medal for his work in the army. In 1919 in recognition of his phenomenal contribution to radiology, the University of Hamburg bestowed a special honor upon Albers-Schönberg by electing him as Ordentlicher – full professor. This was the first full professorship of its kind. He held this tenure until his death.

Albers-Schönberg invented compression diaphragm and other technical innovations. His main book, *Die Röntgentechnik*, which described radiographic techniques, was translated into Italian and Russian and appeared in many editions.

Albers-Schönberg was a tall elegant man, friendly, sincere, and ready to help. He was popular among students by his sense of humor and zest for life.

He died at the age of 56 years, on June 6, 1921 in Hamburg from cardiac failure consequent to pneumonia, leaving directions that the results of his autopsy should be published in the interest of other sufferers. ◆

Christian Ingerslev Baastrup

Painful "Kissing Spine"

B aastrup's disease, known as Morbus Baastrup or kissing spine disease, is a mutual compression of the spinous processes with formation of bridges of closely approximated adjacent lumbar vertebrae. It was described in 1933 by the Danish radiologist, Christian Ingerslev Baastrup, who noticed it on radiological assessment of patients who had pain in the back when standing erect, relieved by bending forward.

Christian Ingerslev Baastrup was born January 24, 1885 in Copenhagen. He was the son of wine merchant Carl Lauritz Baastrup and Christiane Margrethe from the village Ingerslev. He attended Borgerdydskolen in Copenhagen. Christian studied medicine in Copenhagen, graduating with highest

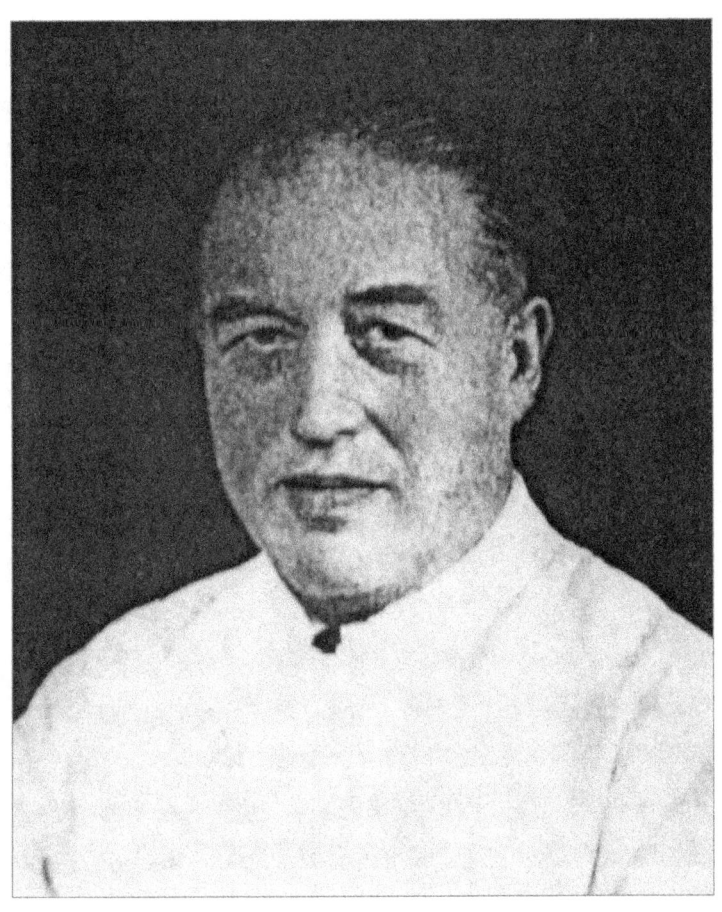

‖ Christian Ingerslev Baastrup*

distinction in 1909. In 1911, after serving as
assistant physician in departments of otolaryngology
and ophthalmology, he was requested to apply for a
position as assistant in the Roentgen department at
Rigshospitalet. He answered the call with a certain
reluctance since at that time, roentgenology did
not enjoy a high esteem in medical circles. His first

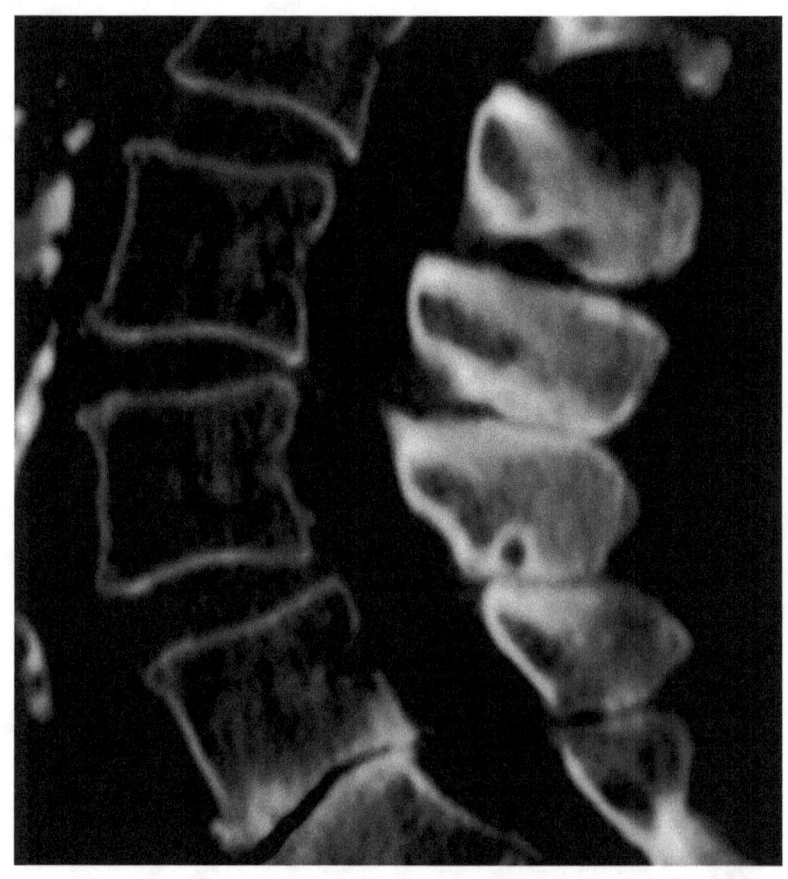

Baastrup disease with close approximation and contact of adjacent spinous processes with resultant enlargement, flattening and reactive sclerosis of interspinous surfaces.

chief and teacher was the prominent roentgenologist H.J.Panner. In 1914, Baastrup was appointed assistant of the genial pioneer J.F.Fischer in the new hospital at Bispebjerg. At Fischer's early death in 1922, Baastrup succeeded him as chief of the department, the most modern in Copenhagen at that time. He was chief of the x-ray clinic from 1922 and was appointed physician-in-chief ("Overlage") in 1935.

Baastrup collaborated in the journal *Acta Radiologica*. He participated in the establishment of the Museum of Medical History of the University of Copenhagen, for which he secured one of the world's largest and most complete collections of x-ray apparatuses. He also invented the Baastrup-Johnsen Roentgen dosimeter.

He was remembered for his quiet, amicable humor and his hospitable home, where he entertained his guests with amusing anecdotes of different countries, having been a great traveler in his younger days.

Christian Baastrup died from cancer of the larynx at the age of 65 on October 24, 1950, at Rigshospitalet, Copenhagen. ◆

Russell Daniel Carman

"A Few Minutes of Screening is Equivalent to Hundreds of Plates"

Carman meniscus sign is a semicircular configuration of gastric ulcer seen in profile with compression. It is suggestive of malignancy.

Russell Daniel Carman was born on March 18, 1875 in Iroquois, Ontario. He was the son of Henry and Sarah (neé Seeley) Carman, both of whom were of prominent United Empire Loyalists descent. The homestead of Carman's ancestors is now a United Empire Loyalist heritage home, known as Carman House Museum, located on 1 Carman Rd, Iroquois, Ontario.

Russell Carman completed his medical courses at Marion Sims College of Medicine in St. Louis, Missouri and received the M.D. degree in 1901. In St. Louis he began a practice in general medicine in partnership with T.Witherspoon. Carman married Sadie L. Butler in 1904 and his partner married Sadie's sister.

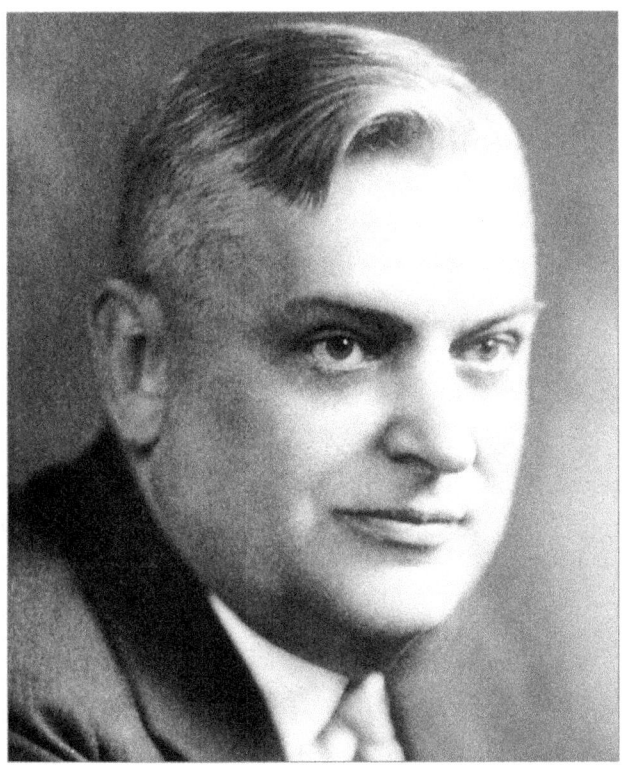

‖ *Russell Daniel Carman**

While practicing general medicine in St. Louis, Carman acquired an x-ray machine early in his practice, and through hard work, he became recognized in the area as an expert in x-ray diagnosis. X-ray tubes in those days contained a small amount of gas necessary for the initial bombardment of the cathode by positive ions to allow the cathode to emit electrons. The function of these tubes was highly unpredictable, and considerable expertise was required for Carman and other pioneers to create a satisfactory x-ray image.

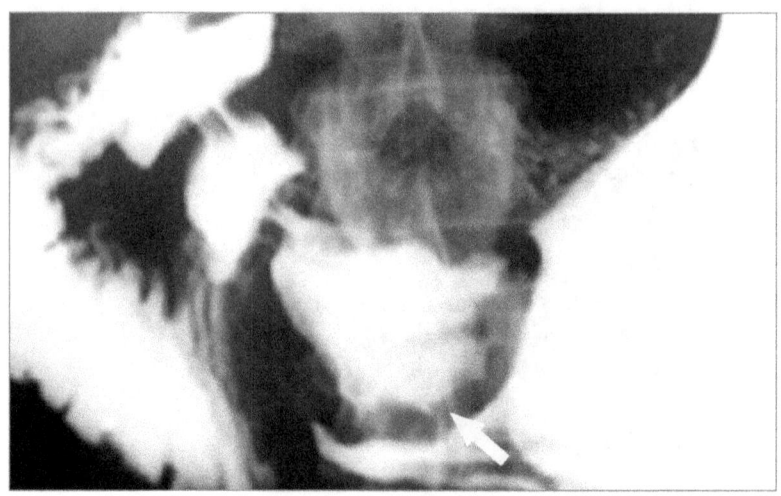

Carman meniscus sign - semicircular configuration of gastric ulcer seen in profile with compression*

Carman was appointed professor of roentgenology at St. Louis University and Washington University Schools of Medicine. In 1913, invited by William J. Mayo, Carman founded the Department of Diagnostic Radiology at the Mayo Clinic and was a head of the Mayo Section on Roentgenology. Carman held that position until his death.

From 1907 to 1917, working with gas tubes, Carman studied and gathered data on the roentgenologic aspects of gastrointestinal diseases. To confirm and correlate his results he regularly attended the operations. Carman believed that "a few minutes of screening is equivalent to hundreds of plates", relying primarily on rapid accurate fluoroscopy with use of manual palpation. In the early

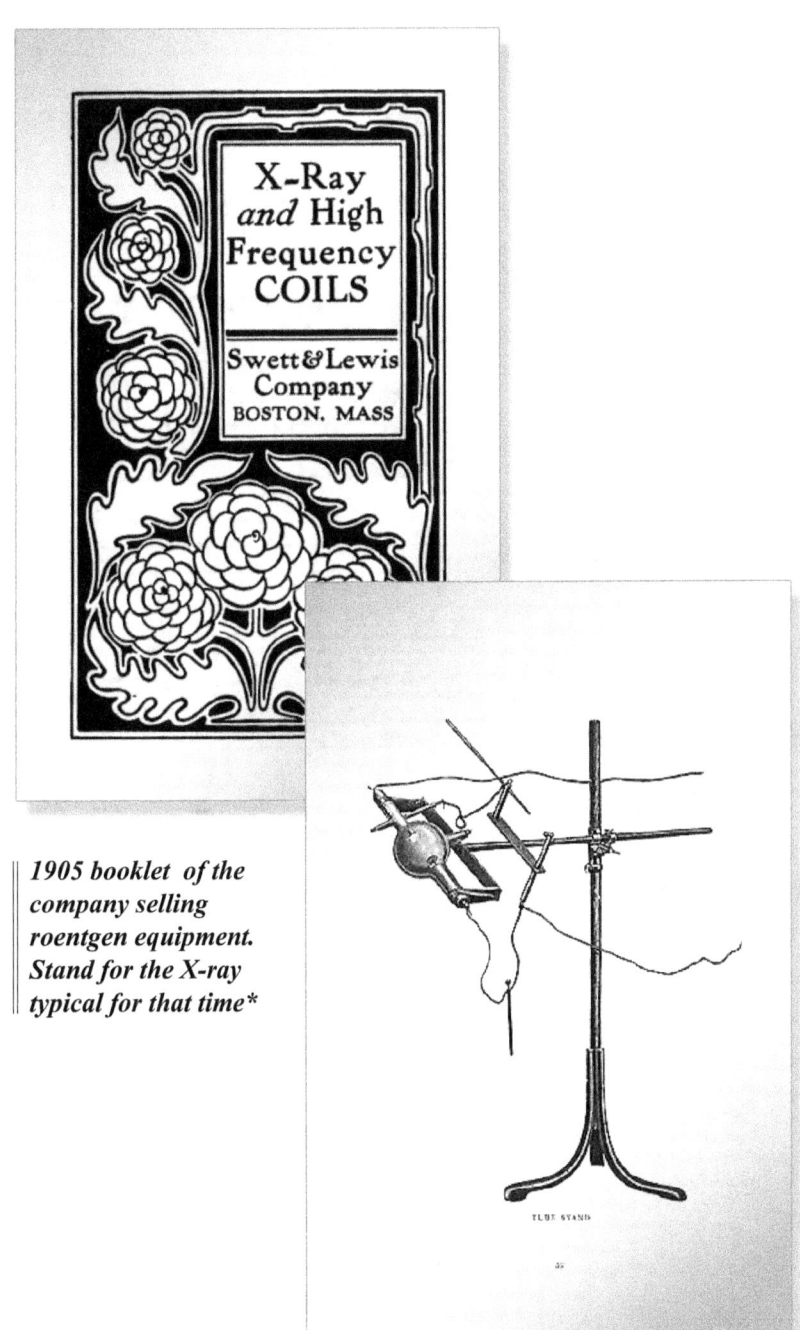

X-Ray
and High
Frequency
COILS

Swett & Lewis
Company
BOSTON, MASS

TUBE STAND

*1905 booklet of the
company selling
roentgen equipment.
Stand for the X-ray
typical for that time**

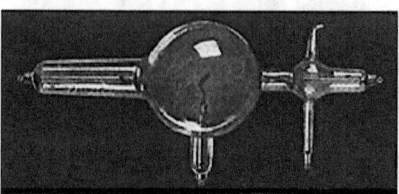

Swett and Lewis Company

X-Ray Tubes

TYPE H. F.

The type H. F. Tube was designed specially for use with high frequency coils, and is a modification of the old Type H, combined with the valve tube so called. The reversed waves are choked back so that the hemispherical effect so familiar to static users is produced. This Tube should be a general favorite, as it is capable of very hard usage. It is recommended for all coils giving an alternating current. The Tube is strongly built, the bulb of good size,

SPECIAL H. F. X-RAY TUBE

and the terminals are well supported, so that they will not break down either in use or during transportation.

Code word, Dejor . . . . Price, $14.00

TYPE K.

This Tube is of good size and shape and is designed for heavy work. The anode is very heavy and is supported on a steel rod. It may be heated to a bright red, and held at this point for a long time without danger of injury to the tube or anode. The definition and penetration are exceptionally good.

The Tube is fitted with a chemical adjustment, which is regulated operated either by heat or spark. If too much gas the anode will be re-absorbed, if the Tube is allowed to rest.

Code word, Delustro . . . . Price, $12.00

Swett and Lewis C

PRICE I

JACKSON HIGH FREQUENCY COIL, to from 52 to 250 volts and any commercia page 4, including electrodes, stand and tul
Code word, Heidengeld.

JACKSON HIGH FREQUENCY COIL for including motor generator . . . .
Code word, Headledge.

JACKSON HIGH FREQUENCY COIL for including motor generator . . . .
Code word, Heenkomen.

MOTOR GENERATOR including starting when sold without coil . . .
Code word, Hervatting.

MOTOR GENERATOR including starting when sold without coil . . .
Code word, Hervimos.

MOTOR GENERATOR including starting when sold without coil . . .
Code word, Hervento.

CAUTERY TRANSFORMER, additional
Code word, Curtelasse.

This transformer put up in fine case, to use separately from coil, $20.00.
Code word, Curtinho.

CAUTERY HANDLE with snare . . . . Price, $6.00
Code word, Curtem.

CAUTERY HANDLE, plain . . . . Price, $1.50
Code word, Curtiamos.

CAUTERY CORDS, per pair . . . . Price, $1.80
Code word, Curtidos.

CAUTERY KNIVES, No. 1 to No. 8 . . . . . Price, each $0.75
See illustration on page 10.
Code word for set of eight, Curtilage.

ULTRA VIOLET ATTACHMENT, including lamp, cable and arm for tube stand . . . . Price, $60.00
Code word, Conjunctam.

COMPRESSOR with fine quartz lens . . . . Price, $5.00
Code word, Condate.

SET OF METALLIC HIGH FREQUENCY ELECTRODES, when sold separately . . . .
Code word, Hervencia.

SET OF SIX GLASS VACUUM ELECTRODES with . . . rice. $5.00
Code word, Koukarsen.

SPECIAL H. F. X-RAY TUBE, as shown on page Price. $14.00
Code word, Depor.

MINERAL TUBES, to be used as electrodes, 20 inches long, ve
Code word, Demram.

$14 and $12 - prices of x-ray tubes at the time of Russell Carman*

years before the perfection of reliable spot films, he also used the orthodiagraphoscope, an apparatus custom-made for him by the Keleket Corporation which allowed the image to be traced on a fluoroscopic screen with a pen and later transferred to the paper.

In collaboration with Albert Miller, a skilled medical writer, Carman published his book "The Roentgen Diagnosis of Diseases of the Alimentary Canal" in 1917. It was the first definitive text on alimentary tract roentgenology and is still an influential reference. In addition to the best known sign of ulcerating carcinoma, which bears his name, he and Miller also described other classic findings such as "hourglass" stomach, the "niche," the "filling defect," and the "incisura."

Carman was extremely friendly, charming, and intelligent. He was interested in cars and in design of x-ray equipment, including a rocker for shaking and drying x-ray plates and a revolving radiographic table that allowed stereoscopic and Bucky diaphragm work.

In September 1925, Carman became ill and underwent fluoroscopy. Films were placed on Carman's desk without comment. He took the images and holding them up to the window stated "cancer of the stomach, inoperable." An hour later, he presented a lecture to 2,600 physicians at the Interstate Postgraduate Assembly of North America. He remained active in the field until his death on June 17, 1926 of the disease for the diagnosis of which he had become famous. ◆

Demetrius Chilaiditi

Success, Mystery and Obscurity

C hilaiditi syndrome is a well known and commonly diagnosed x-ray finding of interposition of a bowel between liver and right diaphragm and may be associated with abdominal pain, vomiting, anorexia, and distension. The man that this syndrome is named after was known as Demetrius Chilaiditi. He was born in Vienna, son of prosperous diasporal Greek Georges Chilaiditi, on April 11, 1883. They lived in the house on prestigious Viennese Favoritenstrasse 45. Demetrius studied at the University of Vienna, graduating in 1908. Fascinated by new and attractive radiology, he went to gain radiological experience working at the III Medical University Clinic in

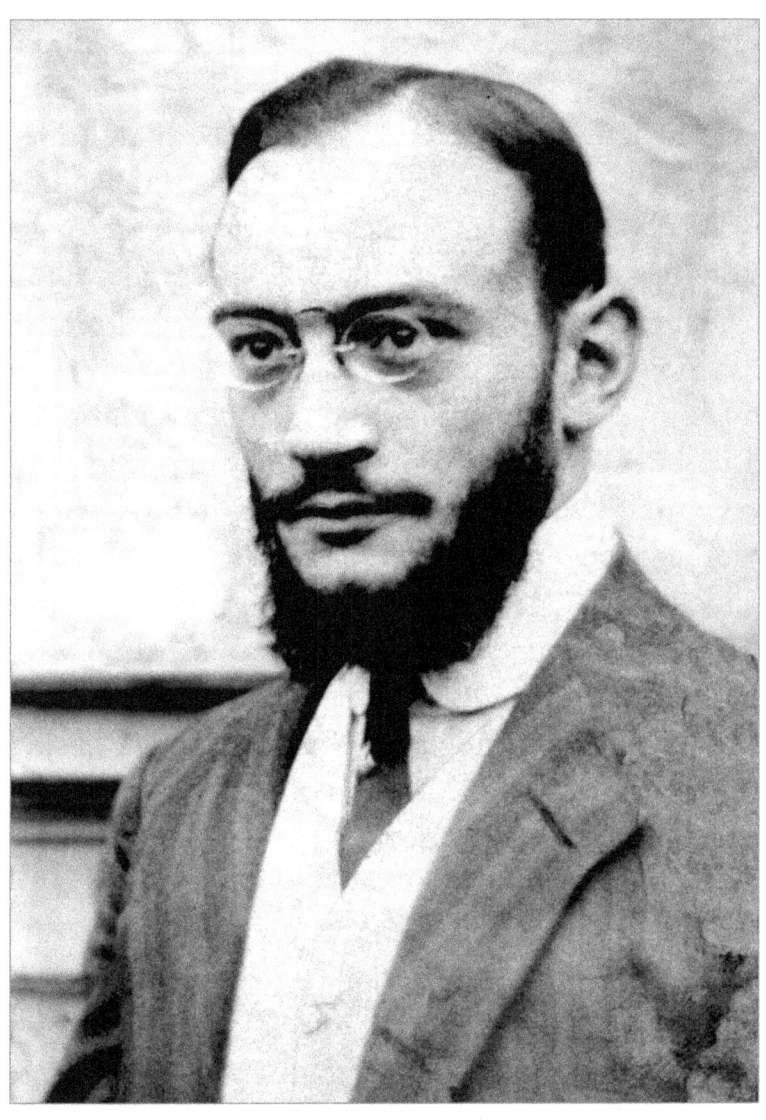

Demetrius Chilaiditi. Previously unpublished photograph from the family archives. Courtesy of Gerry Livadas.

Vienna and at the Zentral-Röntgeninstitut. Among his teachers was Professor Guido Holzknecht who had described retrocardiac space and Robert Kienböck – discoverer of lunatomalacia (known now as Kienböck's disease). Later Chilaiditi mastered his radiology knowledge learning in France under Raoul Bensaude (who described lipomatosis known as the "Launois-Bensaude Syndrome")

In 1910 Chilaiditi came to Constantinople (Istanbul) with large plans and ambitions. However, in Constantinople his path crossed with the activity of another x-ray enthusiast and pioneer. The first x-ray laboratory had been working in Constantinople since 1905. It was run by former Polish ophthalmologist, Albert Englander, who opened his private laboratory in Beyoğlu (then known as Pera - the European side) of Constantinople. Overcoming a lot of difficulties including lack of electrical power in Constantinople of those days, Englander started his career as a radiologist. He had to use a manual dynamo machine to provide electrical power to his x-ray equipment. In 1906 Englander published his radiological findings on cancer therapy by x-rays.

In Constantinople, Chilaiditi became the second radiologist with a private laboratory in the city. He placed his practice in a 2-storey house. He had to overcome the same technical difficulties as Englander. To have electricity connected to the building in

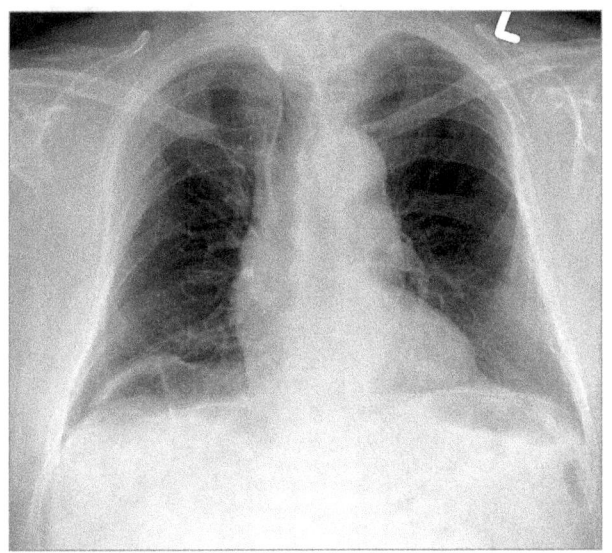

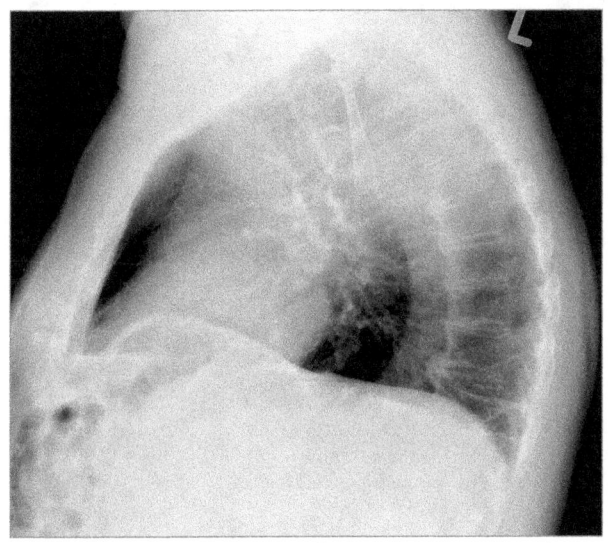

Chilaiditi syndrome - interposition of a bowel between liver and right diaphragm.

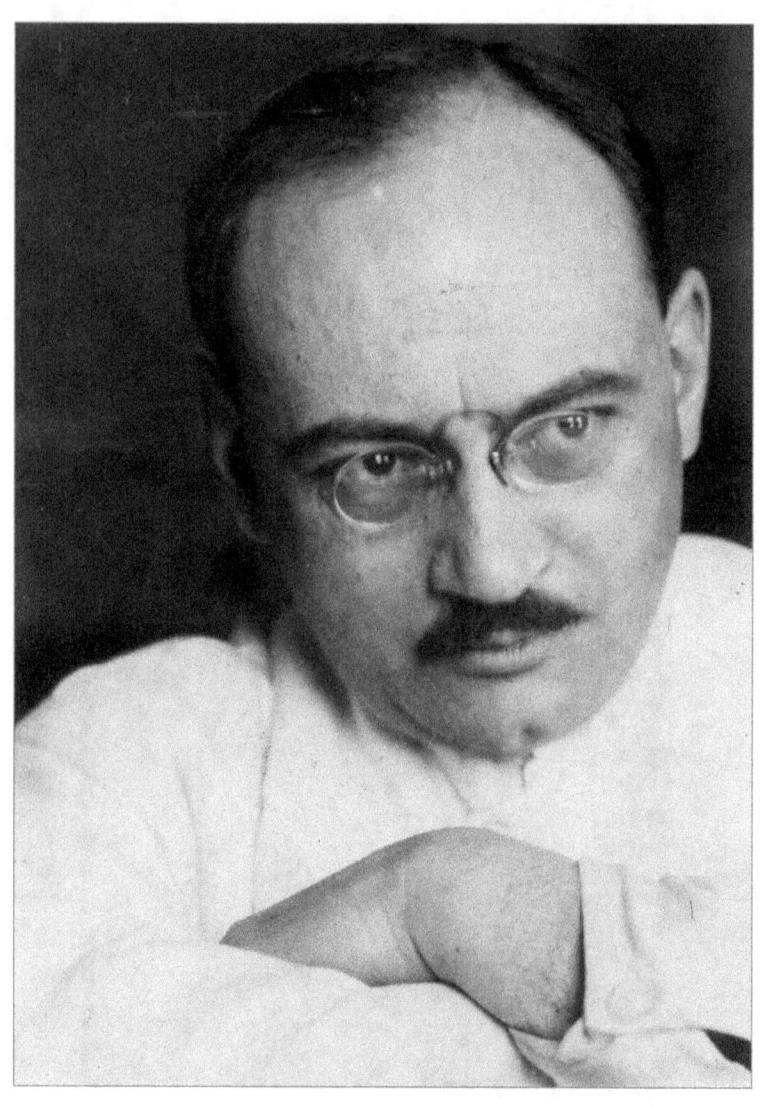

Demetrius Chilaiditi. Previously unpublished photograph from the family archives. Courtesy of Gerry Livadas.

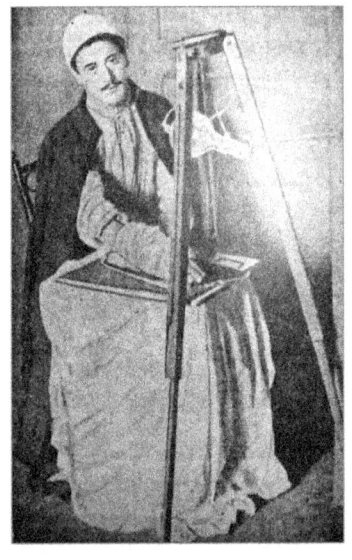

Equipment used to acquire the
x-ray of Turkish soldier in 1897.

Constantinople at that time one needed a special permission. Not being able to get this permission, Chilaiditi hired a Turk worker whose job was to be in the basement and run the dynamo machine. When ready, the worker yelled 'Now!' signalling that Chilaiditi could take an x-ray. Chilaiditi's reputation as a Vienna-educated radiologist, new equipment and personal connections guaranteed lots of referrals from the hospitals and clinics.

The laboratory was so successful that the competition with Englander caused rivalry. Rumors circulated that Englander tried to get rid of Chilaiditi. This plan did not succeed. The sudden disappearance of Englander from the city left no clue. Did he leave to avoid repercussions? Or maybe the then dark streets of Constantinople witnessed one of their mysterious dramas?

Chilaiditi also worked as a radiologist at the French, Greek, and Italian hospitals in Constantinople. Until 1936 he served as the chairman of the Radiology

Department of the English hospital in Constantinople while at the same time continuing to run his private practice. His early retirement was attributed to the radiation related complications.

Chilaiditi became one of the first members of the Turkish Radiological Society.

In his work, published in 1910, Demetrius Chilaiditi reported on the anatomo-radiographic aspects of three asymptomatic cases of the appearance of subdiaphragmatic air on plain radiography due to temporary hepato-diaphragmatic interposition of the colon. Bowel interposition is caused by congenital anomalies of the falciform ligament of the diaphragm. Some patients complained of a feeling of pressure on the upper part of the belly, which recedes when lying down.

The phenomenon of interposition of the intestine between the liver and the diaphragm was first described by Cantini in 1865. In 1899 Béclère presented the necropsy and roentgenological findings in a patient thought to have a subdiaphragmatic abscess.

Since its publication by Chilaiditi this condition has been associated with his name.

Chilaiditi published almost 90 works on the radiotherapy of malignant tumors, hypertrichosis, gynecological diseases and duodenal stenosis. Chilaiditi spoke fluent Turkish, Greek, German and French. *The British Medical Journal* in 1911 reported about the attention drawn by Societe de Radiologie Medicale de Paris when Demetrius Chilaiditi suggested that pyloric function and acid-base was involved in duodenal diseases including ulcer.

Chilaiditi's son, George, named according to Greek tradition after his grandfather worked in Athens as a gastroenterologist. In 1950s he was tried for his Communist activities. He died in a car accident. Chilaiditi's grandchildren, Irini and Demetrius, live in London and Athens. Demetrius Chilaiditi's great-grandson is a radiologist in Great Britain. Though having tight family and friendship connections to Greece, Demetrius Chilaiditi did not move to live there staying with his second wife, who was Turkish. He died in Istanbul on January 2, 1975.

The differences in the spelling of Demetrius Chilaiditi's last name can cause some confusion. The Greek spelling of the name is ΚΗΛΑΙΔΙΤΗΣ. In modern Greek "H" sounds like "I" and becomes "I", the Greek "K" becomes "Ch", transforming ΚΗΛΑΙΔΙΤΗΣ into Chilaiditis in accordance with traditional Greek pronunciation of the name (therefore, Chilaiditi syndrome is frequently pronounced as Chilaiditis). It is commonly written as Khlaidiths or Kelaiditis. Some of Demetrius Chilaiditi's descendents spell their last name as Kilaiditi. ◆

Ernest Amory Codman

Ostracism and Fame

Codman Triangle is a pattern seen in rapidly growing bone processes such as neoplasms, particularly osteosarcoma and osteomyelitis. When a process is growing too fast for the periosteum to respond with even thin shells of new bone, sometimes only the edges of the raised periosteum will ossify. A localized, triangular ridge of new bone is formed where periosteum is elevated. The sign was described by Boston surgeon E. A. Codman.

Ernest Amory Codman was born on December 30, 1869 in Boston, MA. He belonged to the First Families of Boston (also called Boston Brahmins - the class of descendants from the English Protestants who founded the city and settled New England). Codman graduated from Harvard Medical School in 1895

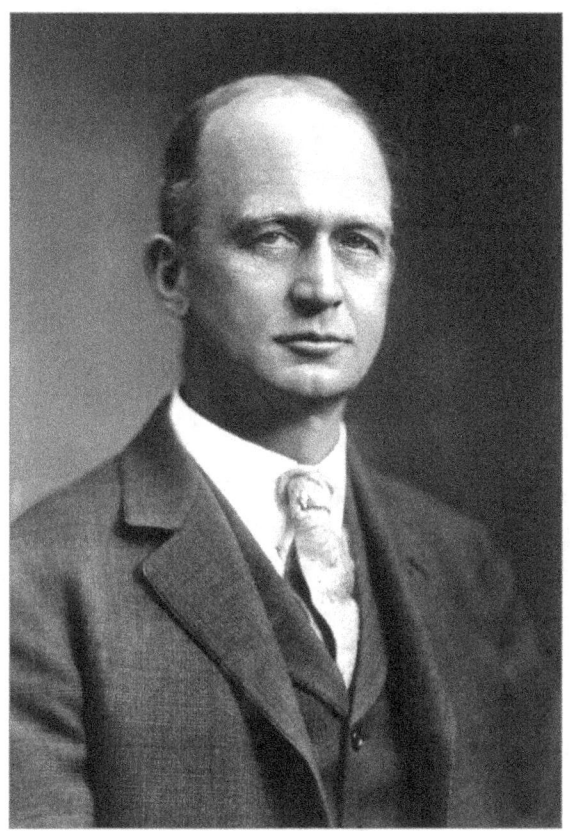

Ernest Amory Codman*

and completed his internship at the Massachusetts General Hospital. He became a member of the Harvard Faculty and was a founder of the American College of Surgeons. He lost his staff privileges in 1914 when the hospital refused to institute his plan for evaluating the competence of surgeons.

In 1915 Codman was ostracised and ordered to step down as Chair of the surgical society for public

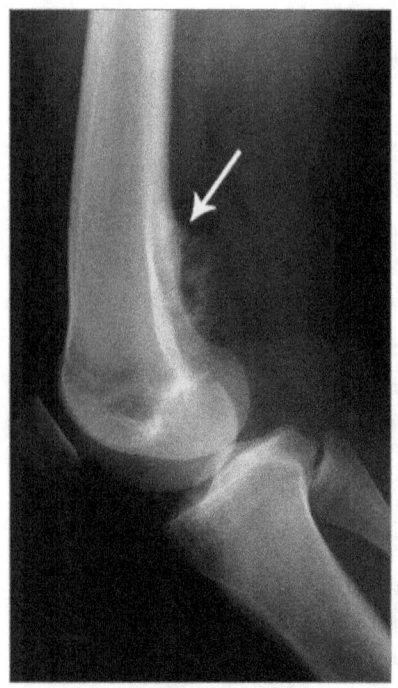

Codman triangle - a localized, triangular ridge of new bone is formed where periosteum is elevated in rapidly growing bone processes such as neoplasms, particularly osteosarcoma and osteomyelitis*

insult by his colleagues after he presented a large cartoon at a meeting of the local surgical society which he chaired, which portrayed greedy surgeons grasping for gold from wealthy patients (shown as an ostrich with its head buried in Boston's prosperous Beacon Hill).

Codman is famous for his lifelong systematic effort to follow up each of his patients years after treatment and to record the end results of their care. He established the first bone tumor registry in the United States in the 1920s and set the precedent for a national exchange of information on bone tumors.

Codman said that most clinical research described

only very good results and were therefore mere advertisements. He believed that real improvement would be made when clinicians wrote about their errors and how to reduce them.

On December 7, 1917, the day after the munitions ship explosion in Halifax, Nova Scotia which killed 3000 and injured 20000 people, Codman closed his hospital and left to help to care for victims.

Codman made important contributions to surgery including his privately printed in 1934 book, "The Shoulder", the first medical book on this topic.

Ernest Amory Codman died on November 23, 1940 in Ponkapoag, MA. ◆

Christian Andreas Doppler

Struggle, Mistake and Discovery

D oppler effect, a change in the frequency of light and sound waves, is related to the velocity of the source relative to an observer. It is used in sonography to estimate the blood flow.

Christian Doppler (on his baptismal certificate Christian Andreas Doppler, on his gravesite Christian Johann Doppler) was born November 29, 1803 in Salzburg, Austria. To earn his living, Doppler worked as a bookkeeper at a cotton-spinning factory. Having decided to immigrate to America, he sold all he had to finance his journey. He later cancelled his plans and stayed in Austria waiting for two years to get the post at the Technical Secondary School in Prague in 1835. For five years he applied for a position as professor of higher mathematics at the Polytechnic in Prague but

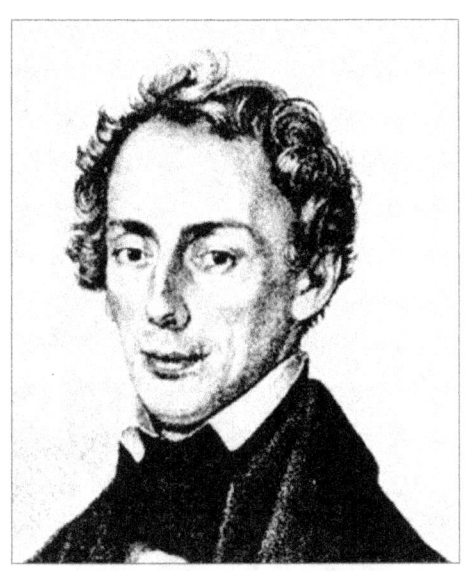

|| *Christian Doppler*

without success. Only in 1841 was he appointed to this post. Doppler's students complained that he was too harsh in his examining. Doppler was investigated and reprimanded while the students were allowed to retake their examinations.

Having a difficult time in Prague, Doppler moved to a professorship of mathematics, physics and mechanics at the Academy of Mines and Forests in Banska Stiavnica. As a result of the stormy revolutionary year of 1848, Doppler sought refuge, finding it at the Vienna Polytechnic. On January 17, 1850 he was appointed as the first director of the new Institute of Physics at Vienna University reaching the highest point of his career. Just after Doppler's dreams came true, his health deteriorated. In November

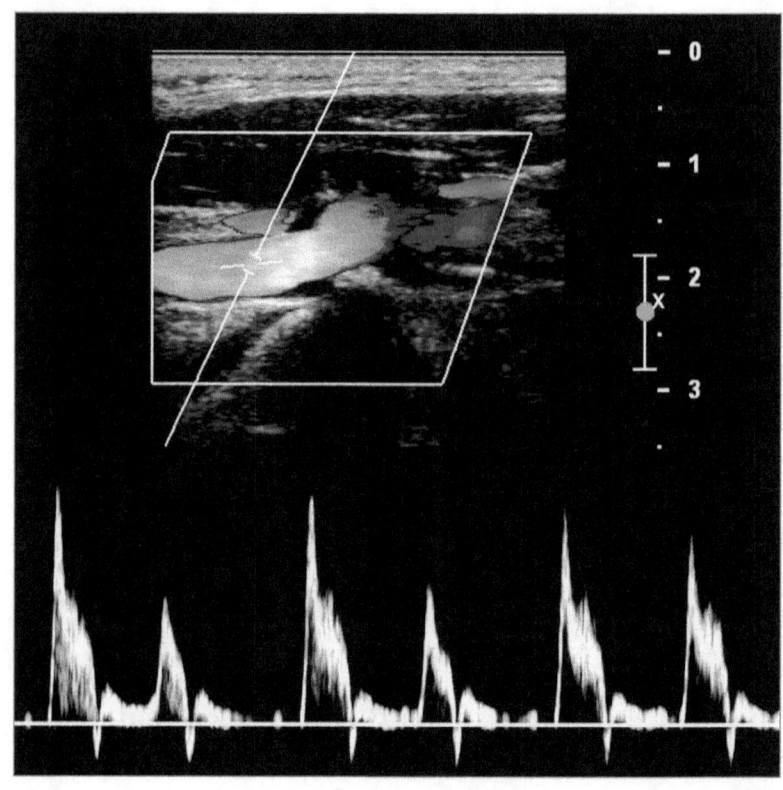

Doppler effect used to assess blood flow on ultrasound.

1852, he traveled to Venice, Italy and died there a few months later on March 17, 1853.

Doppler had difficulty becoming a member of the Royal Bohemian Society. Only after he introduced his most famous of ideas to the Royal Bohemian Society in 1842, was he elected as an ordinary member of the Society. On May 25, 1842, Doppler presented the paper "On the coloured light of the double stars and certain other stars of the heavens". The paper described what came to be known for the first time as the Doppler principle which relates the frequency of a source to its velocity relative to an observer. Doppler derived the principle in a few lines treating both light and sound as longitudinal waves in the ether and matter, respectively.

Interestingly, Doppler was incorrect regarding light being a longitudinal wave. He also was wrong when he tried to illustrate his theory with an application to the colors of double stars - the effect is too small to be significant.

However, the situation with sound was different. In 1845 experiments were conducted with musicians on railway trains playing instruments and other trained musicians writing down the apparent note as the train approached and then receded from them. In 1846 Doppler published a better version of his principle where he considered both the motion of the source and the motion of the observer. Doppler had many new ideas which led to many inventions, particularly of optical instruments and to improvement of existing ones. ◆

Felix George Fleischner
Doyen of Radiodiagnosis

Fleischner lines are horizontal dense lines of atelectasis and healed infarction, often seen in the lower lung fields and vary from barely visible lines to shadows of about 5 mm in thickness. They are usually located about 1 to 3 cm above the dome of the diaphragm.

Fleischner sign is a prominent central artery which can be caused either by pulmonary hypertension that develops secondary to peripheral embolization or by distention of the vessel by a large clot.

These were described by Felix George Fleischner, an Austrian and American radiologist.

He was born in Vienna on July 29, 1893. Fleischner graduated from the University of Vienna Medical School. After training in radiology he became

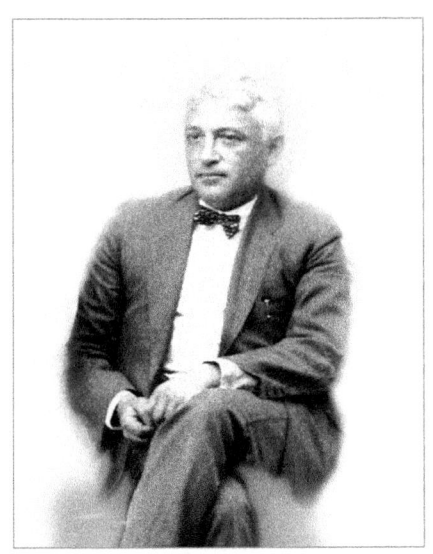

Felix George Fleischner.
Original photo made in Vienna
in 1925. From the inheritance of
*Guido Holzknecht**

chief of the roentgen department of the Vienna CS
Child's Hospital. In 1930 he became Professor and
head of radiology of the Second Medical Clinic of the
University.

Before World War II Fleischner had published 87
papers. He was recognized as a renowned lecturer in
radiology of the post-graduate courses sponsored by
the University of Vienna and the American Medical
Association.

In 1938, following the annexation of Austria by
Hitler on March 11, 1938 and subsequent eviction of
Jews from Vienna University, Dr. Fleischner decided

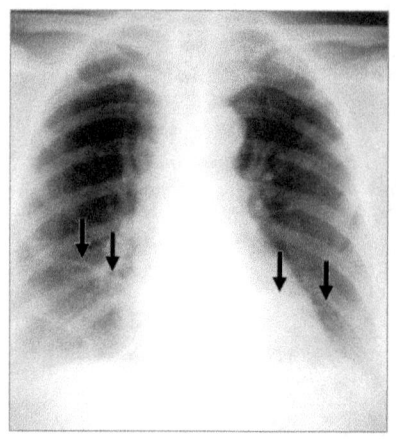

to leave. On August
30, 1938, accompanied
by his wife Risa and
daughters, Susanne and
Elisabeth, he came to New York on board the SS *Ile
de France*. They headed to Boston where they were
met by Flieschner's friend, Eric Pick. In Boston,
Fleischner worked in the radiology department of
the Massachusetts General Hospital and in private
practice in Greenfield, Massachusetts.

In 1942 he got a position at Beth Israel Hospital
with appointments at Harvard and Tufts Medical
Schools. Fleischner started the first formal residency
training program in radiology at BIH, and became
Professor of Radiology at Harvard in 1952. He
strongly emphasised the value of radiologic teaching
and research.

Working in the United States, Fleischner
published an additional 165 scientific articles. He
received many honors. Two international symposia,
the first on pulmonary embolism and the second
on frontiers of chest radiology, were dedicated to

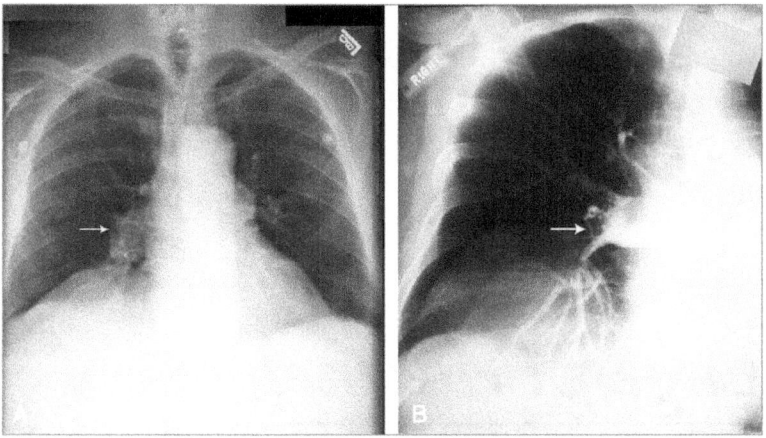

Fleischner sign - Enlargement of the right interlobar artery (arrow). The follow-up angiogram confirms the presence of filling defects representing multiple emboli and a distended right interlobar artery*

him. Interestingly, in 1965 at the 600th anniversary of the University of Vienna, Fleischner represented the Harvard Medical School. Fleischner retired from Beth Israel Hospital in 1960; however, he continued teaching at the Peter Bent Brigham Hospital and the Massachusetts General Hospital until his death.

Felix Fleischner died on August 17, 1969 in Boston – a few months before the inaugural meeting of a new multidisciplinary international society of leading experts in chest disease he had been invited to attend. The greatest memorial tribute was the adoption of his name by this prestigious society – now Fleischner Society. ◆

Eugen Fraenkel

From Ophthalmology to Fame in Pathology and Bacteriology

Fraenkel line - white line of metaphyseal zone of preparatory calcification in cases of infantile scurvy.

Eugen Fraenkel was born on September 28, 1853 in the city of Neustadt, Silesia. He was descended from a family of famous Jewish scholars and Talmudists which followed its roots from Vienna. His father was a physician, Dr. Wolff (Wilhelm) Fraenkel (1826-1901), and mother Johanna Haase (1833-1908), was the daughter of the owner of a tannery. Eugen Fraenkel studied at the University of Vienna. He completed medical studies in Breslau in 1874. Fraenkel started

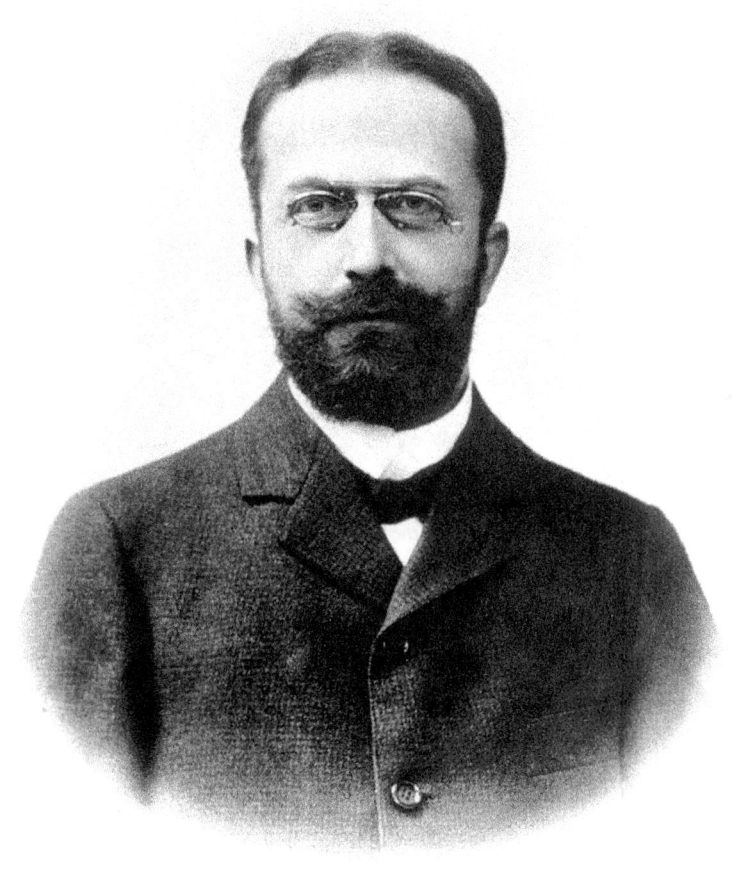

|| *Eugen Fraenkel**

his medical career in Hamburg as an assistant at the ophthalmic clinic of St. Georg Hospital.

In 1879 he switched from ophthalmology to pathology. Fame came to Fraenkel who demonstrated

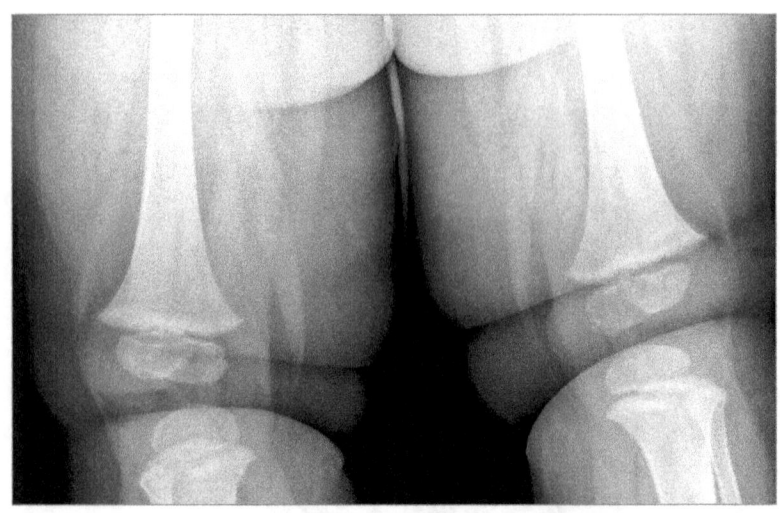

Fraenkel line - white line of metaphyseal zone of preparatory calcification in cases of infantile scurvy*

pathogenic properties of typhoid fever bacilli and published the book in 1886. In 1889 Fraenkel moved to the new Institute of Pathology at Eppendorfer Hospital (Eppendorfer Krankenhaus) affiliated with the University of Hamburg and worked there until 1924. At the outbreak of the cholera epidemic in Hamburg in 1892, Eugen Fraenkel was summoned back from his vacation and confirmed the presence of almost pure cholera vibrio in patient's stool.

Fraenkel's greatest discovery was the isolation of primary infective agent in most cases of gas gangrene in 1892. The following year Fraenkel wrote the first monograph on anaerobic wound infection which was consulted as standard during World War I. The gas gangrene bacillus was called initially Bacillus Fraenkel and later renamed Clostridium perfringens.

In 1909, the Senate of Hamburg granted him the rank of Professor. In 1913 Fraenkel was elected president of the "Deutsche Pathologische Gesellschaft" - German Pathological Society. In 1919 Fraenkel became the first person at Hamburg University to be appointed Ordentlicher – full professor of Pathology. He retired in 1924. Fraenkel was an author of 228 publications.

Fraenkel introduced new methods of bacteriology and x-rays into pathological anatomy. He left works on scurvy (Möller-Barlow disease), congenital syphilis, and lymphoma. He wrote "The Atlas of Normal and Pathologic Anatomy in Typical X-ray Images".

Fraenkel was described as markedly factual to the point of gruffness, taciturn, distrustful and initially critical to everything new. In a word, he was one not to be influenced. His custom was to speak abruptly and briskly. He was unshakable. He could say "I see what you mean. But you can't convince me that it is really so."

Since October 5, 1880, Eugene Fraenkel was married to Marie Deutsch (1861-1943). They had three children – Max, Hans and Margarete.

Eugene Fraenkel died in Hamburg on December 19, 1925.

The rise of Nazism in 1930s heavily affected Fraenkel's family. Marie Fraenkel perished in the Theresienstadt concentration camp in 1943. Max, a physician in Hamburg, committed suicide under pressure of anti-semitic chicanery. Margarete was killed during the last gassing at Auschwitz-Birkenau concentration camp. Hans left Germany to work as an economist and journalist in Switzerland. His descendants are living in Switzerland and Italy. ◆

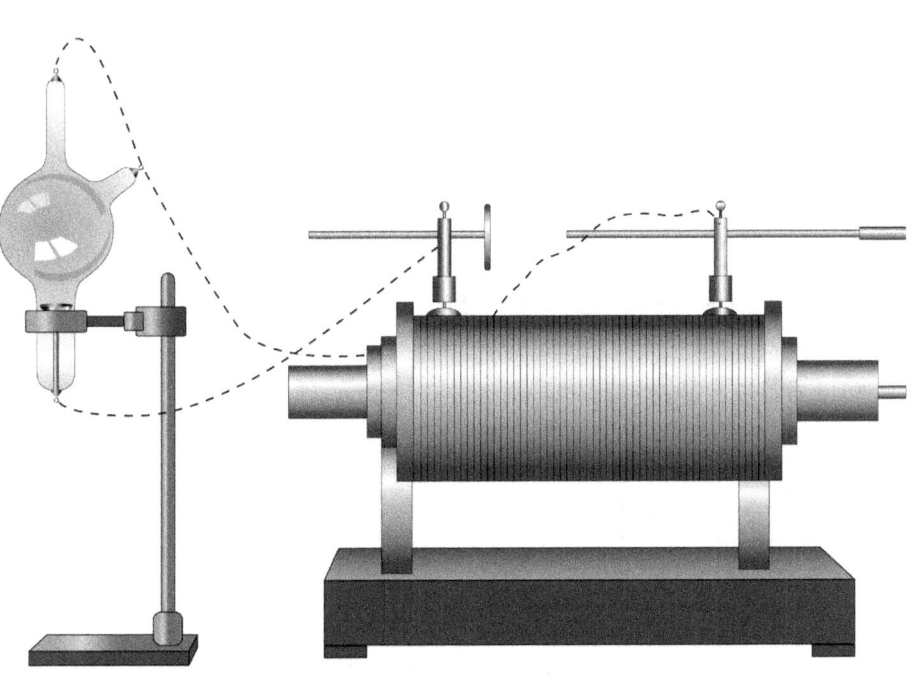

X-RAY APPARATUS OF 1896.
THIS WAS A BEGINNING.
ALL FUTURE DEVELOPMENTS WERE BASED ON
IMPROVEMENTS OF THESE BASIC COMPONENTS.

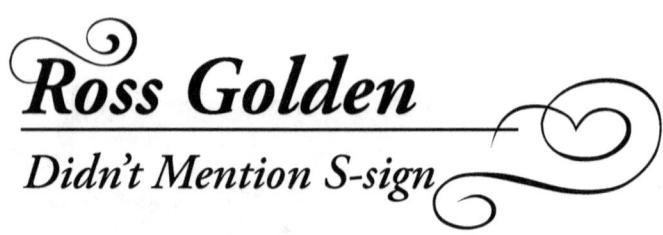

Ross Golden
Didn't Mention S-sign

Golden sign is an elevation and medial displacement of the minor fissure with proximal convexity of the fissure and creation of the "reverse S"- a form of right upper lobe collapse associated with right upper lobe bronchus obstruction.

Ross Golden was born in Iowa Center, Iowa on September 30, 1889 into the family of a Methodist minister. He died in California on January 10, 1975. Golden was a member of the baseball and football teams in Manning High School, Manning, Iowa. After graduating from Harvard Medical School he served in France in WWI. Golden was one of the very first students to go through the original radiology residency program at the Massachusetts General Hospital. He worked at the Presbyterian Hospital

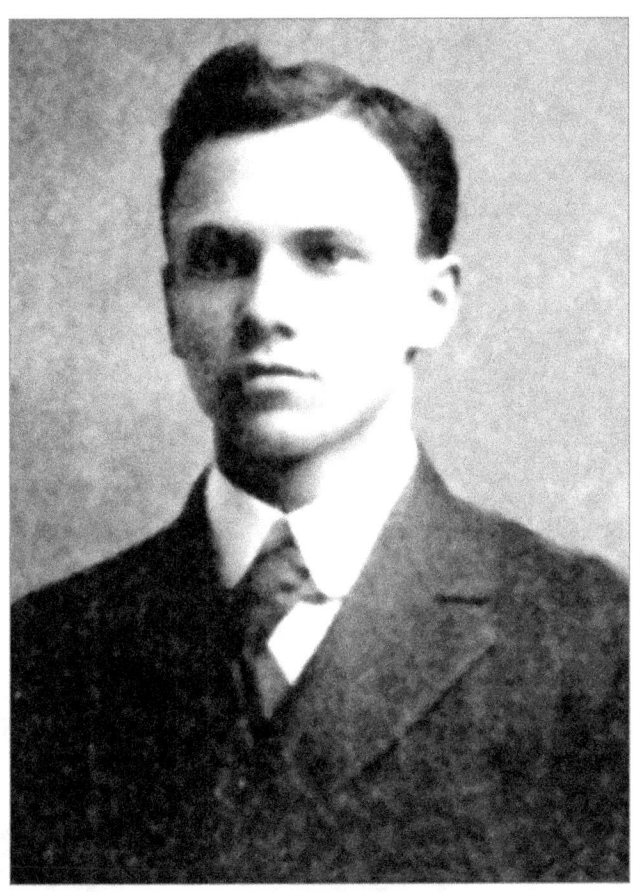

Ross Golden

in New York on the faculty of Columbia University Medical School.

At that time he published the work which made his name famous. He described five cases of bronchial invasion by cancer. Two cases (cases III and V) described tumors obstructing the right upper lobe bronchus with resultant shadow with sharply defined

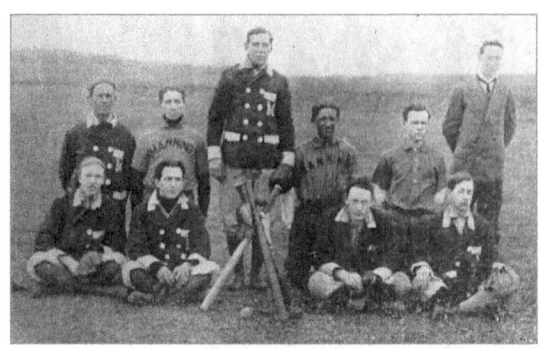

Ross Golden and his baseball team of Manning High School*

concave lower margin. Later the lower margin of the shadow bulged downward and progressed to convex with concave portion located towards the periphery. He did not mention the resemblance of the margin of this shadow to a reverse S. In fact, we were unable to

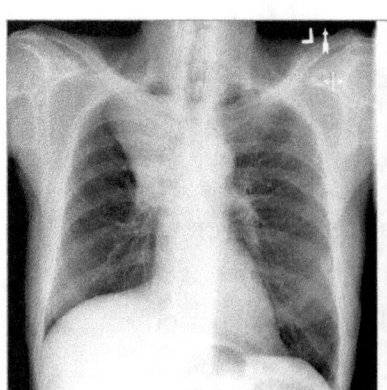 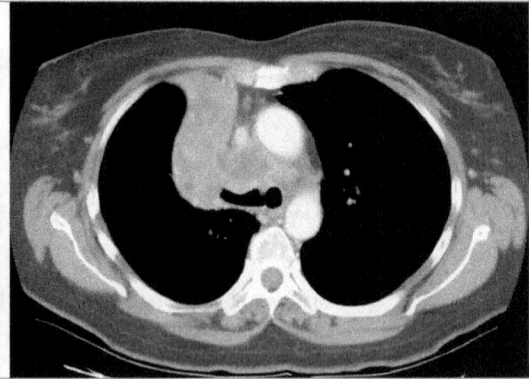

Golden sign - elevation and medial displacement of the minor fissure with proximal convexity of the fissure*

trace who was the first to introduce the term "reverse S sign". In 1927 Golden went to Vienna to take classes from distinguished radiologists. L. Rigler (Rigler sign) was taking the same classes with Golden.

Ross Golden wrote chapters on the roentgen diagnosis of diseases of the small intestine. He helped to organize the American College of Radiology and was a president of the American Roentgen Ray Society. Retiring in 1954 from Columbia, Golden worked for more than 10 years at UCLA where the departmental library was established as the Ross Golden Room.

Ross Golden was known for his intolerance of incompetence, indifference and indolence.

The year of birth of Ross Golden in the memoriam published in Radiology in 1975 is incorrect. ◆

Aubrey Otis Hampton

Liking the Uniform, Abhorring Systematic Teaching

Hampton hump is a pleural-based shallow wedge-shaped consolidation in the lung periphery seen in pulmonary embolism.

Hampton line is a thin, well defined lucent line at the base of the ulcer, reflecting the undermining of the submucosa with preservation of the relatively resistant mucosa.

Aubrey Otis Hampton was born in 1900 in Copeville, Texas. Hampton graduated from Baylor University Medical School, Texas in 1925. He did his radiological training at the Massachusetts General Hospital in Boston. Several years later, he was appointed their Chief of the Department of

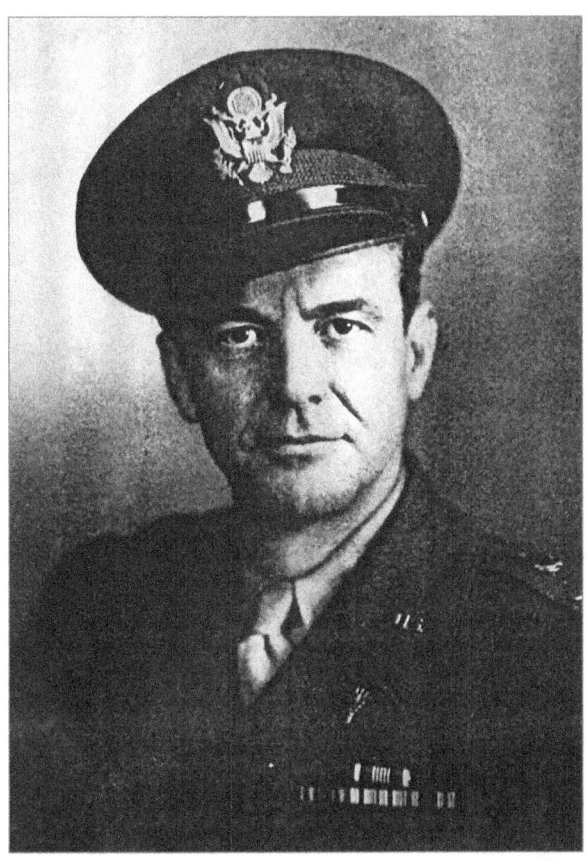

‖ *Aubrey Otis Hampton**

Radiology. During World War II, he stayed stateside as Chief of the Department of Radiology at the Walter Reed Army Hospital, Washington, DC. After the war he was appointed Chief Consultant in Radiology to the Medical Director of the Veteran Administration. Hampton was responsible for creation of a Fellowship for Radiological Pathology at the Armed Forces Institute of Pathology.

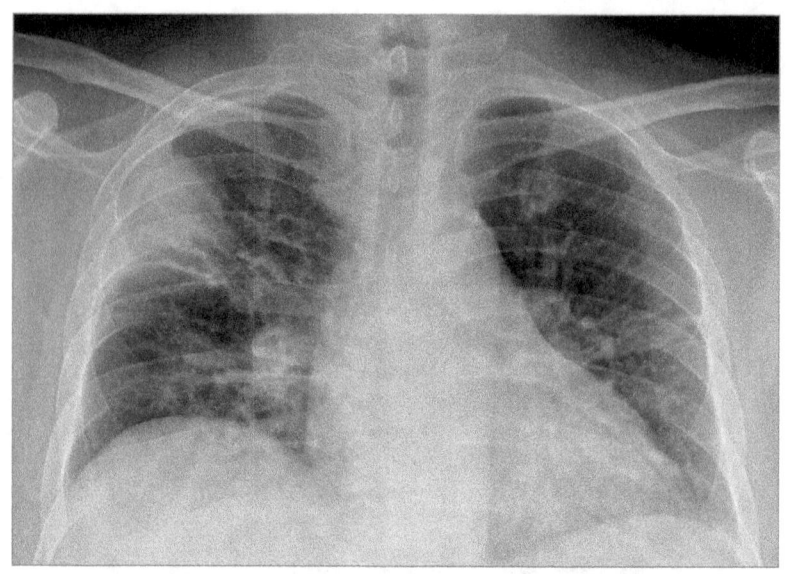

Hampton hump - a peripheral opacity overlying the lateral aspect of the right lung caused by infarction due to pulmonary embolus.

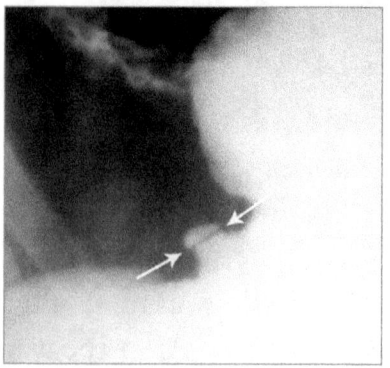

Hampton line - a thin, well defined lucent line at the base of the ulcer, reflecting the undermining of the submucosa with preservation of the relatively resistant mucosa*

Aubrey Hampton was probably one of the most intuitive radiologists of his time. People who worked with Hampton noted that he abhorred systematic and didactic teaching. He used to skip the explanations of preliminary reasons for making a diagnosis, leaving to others to find out why he had made his decision. However, the accuracy of his diagnoses was so high that even this challenge was educational.

Hampton was at his best as a clinical radiologist in the daily routine. His innumerable clinical friends made him the center of their investigating teams. His independent approach to every case was constantly stimulating. His students learned from him to think independently rather than to depend entirely on text book wisdom. He was a man of unusual charm. He made friends easily and kept them. Illness made his last years of life difficult and his early death came as a relief to him. Aubrey Otis Hampton died on July 17, 1955. ◆

Godfrey Newbold Hounsfield

Revolution in Imaging without Background Knowledge in Medicine and Roentgenology

Hounsfield line is a beam hardening artifact seen as an increased attenuation of the x-ray beam due to the density and thickness of the bone.

The Hounsfield unit scale is a quantitative measure of radiodensity used in evaluating CT scans.

Sir Godfrey Newbold Hounsfield was born in Sutton-on-Trent, near Newark in Nottinghamshire on August 28, 1919. He grew up on a farm liking to experiment with the farm's mechanical and electrical machinery. Hounsfield was educated at Magnus Grammar School in Newark-on-Trent having excelled in physics and arithmetic. He always had an aptitude

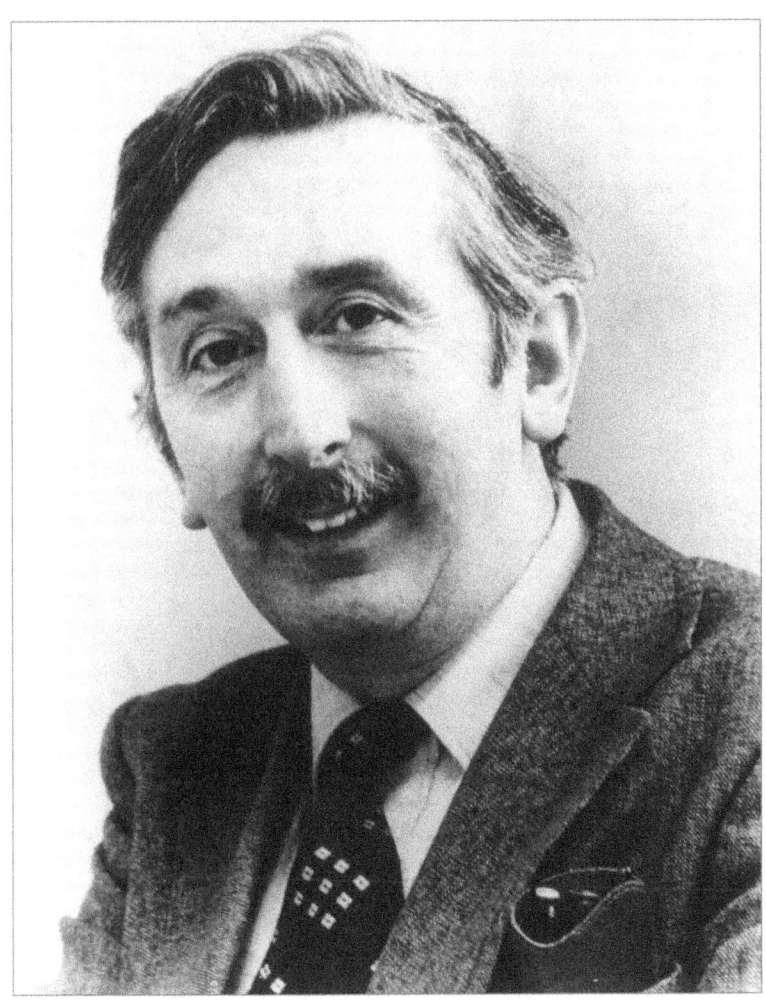

Sir Godfrey Newbold Hounsfield*

for physics and mathematics but never entered a university. After leaving school he worked in a builder's drawing office. Shortly before World War II he joined the Royal Air Force as a volunteer reservist. There he learned the basics of electronics and radar, reading

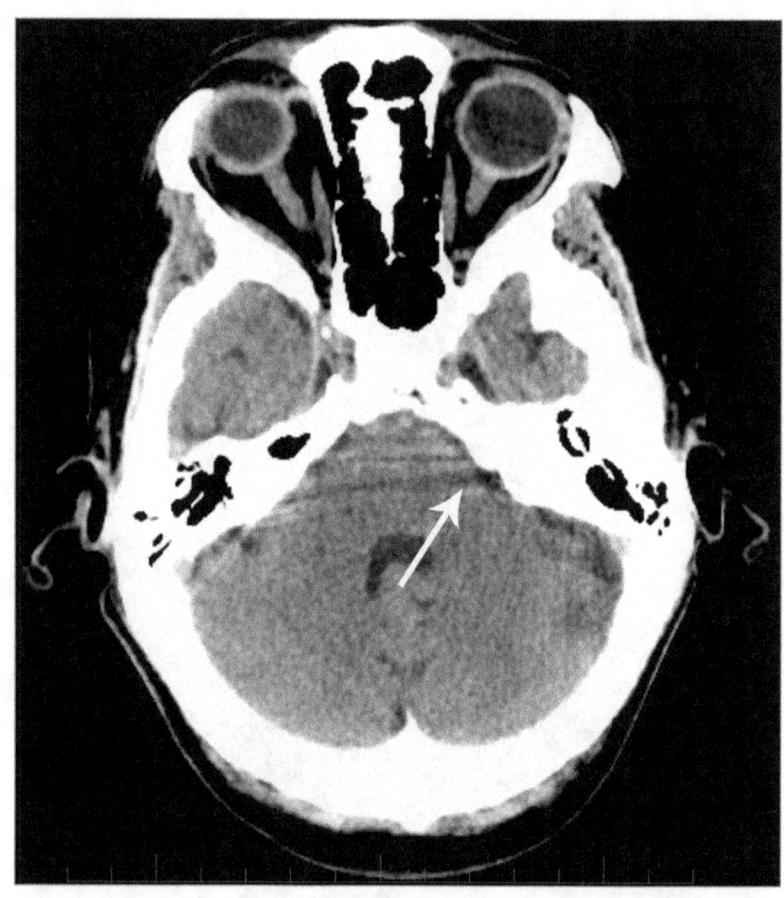

Hounsfield artifact - beam hardening artifact – increased attenuation of the x-ray beam due to the density and thickness of the bone.

some RAF books on radio mechanics, and took a test. He was posted as a radar-mechanic instructor to RAF Cranwell where he was promoted to Corporal. After studying radio communication he passed the City and Guilds examination.

With the help of Air Vice-Marshal J.Cassidy,

Hounsfield obtained a grant which enabled him to attend Faraday House College of Electrical Engineering in London graduating with a Diploma of Faraday House.

In 1951 Hounsfield joined Electrical and Musical Industries (EMI) where he worked on improving radar systems and then on computers. He helped complete production of Britain's first large all-transistor computer in 1959, worked on high-capacity computer memory devices, and was granted a British patent in 1967 for "Magnetic Films for Information Storage".

Hounsfield's work in this period included the problem of enabling computers to recognize patterns, thus allowing them to "read" letters and numbers.

Once, while traveling in the countryside, as he usually liked to do, Hounsfield had his flash of inspiration. He was thinking about his radar research, in particular the problems of pattern recognition. Radar systems scan their surroundings by sending out radio waves from a central point and detecting patterns in the periphery. Why not try the reverse process, Hounsfield thought while walking, and study the central or interior pattern of an object from outside? Why not send beams through a box with unknown number of items inside and, by taking readings at all angles through it, find out what is hidden inside?

He thought to take these readings and then reconstruct in 3-D the content of the box seeing a three-dimensional object as a series of cross-sectional slices.

He then realised that the skull as a box, collimated x-ray beams and computer technology provided the ideal combination. Without any background knowledge in medicine and roentgenology, and being unaware of the equations of variations of body tissues which had been developed by American physicist Allan M. Cormack, Hounsfield envisioned a medical diagnostic system in which radiation source and radiation detector would image thin "slices" through the patient's body and a computer would process the slices into an accurate representation. Hounsfield's research proposal to EMI was entitled "An improved form of X-radiography".

Looking at practical applications of the technique, EMI and Hounsfield approached the British Department of Health and Social Security in London. They asked the Medical Research Council for development funds in exchange for a share of the profits. The government thought that it would be commendable foresight and agreed to support EMI's development of the scanner.

Hounsfield was introduced to C.Gregory, scientific adviser and to C.E.Lennon, a radiological advisor to the Department of Health. One of the

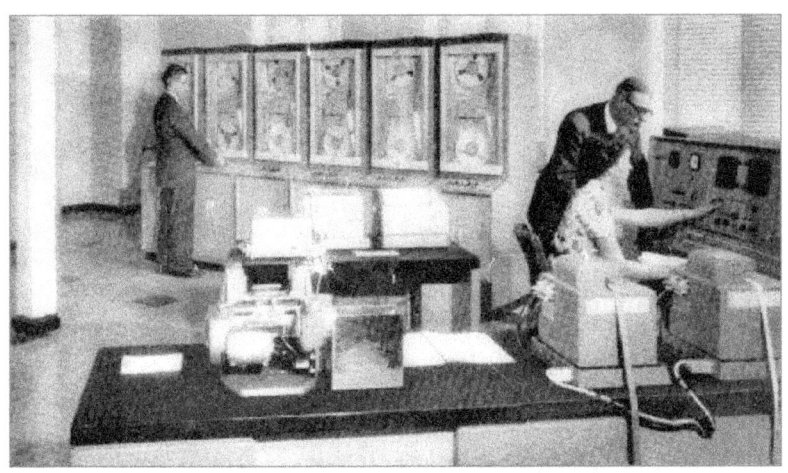

The first commercially available in
Great Britain all-transistor computer
EMIDEC 1100 produced under the
leadership of G.Hounsfield.

eminent radiologists, the first to be invited to meet Hounsfield, dismissed Hounsfield as a crank. However, C.E.Lennon arranged another meeting of Hounsfield, this time with James Ambrose – neuroradiologist from Atkinson Morley's Hospital, Frank Doyle – radiologist from the Hammersmith Hospital and Louis Kreel – radiologist from the Royal Free Hospital. Although Ambrose, who had presented the work on cranial ultrasound and was aware of its limitations seemed to be well prepared to understand Hounsfield's novel ideas, the first meeting did not go well. Ambrose found Hounsfield a difficult character, not very talkative, wary of explaining any details of his invention. Hounsfield responded to all the newest

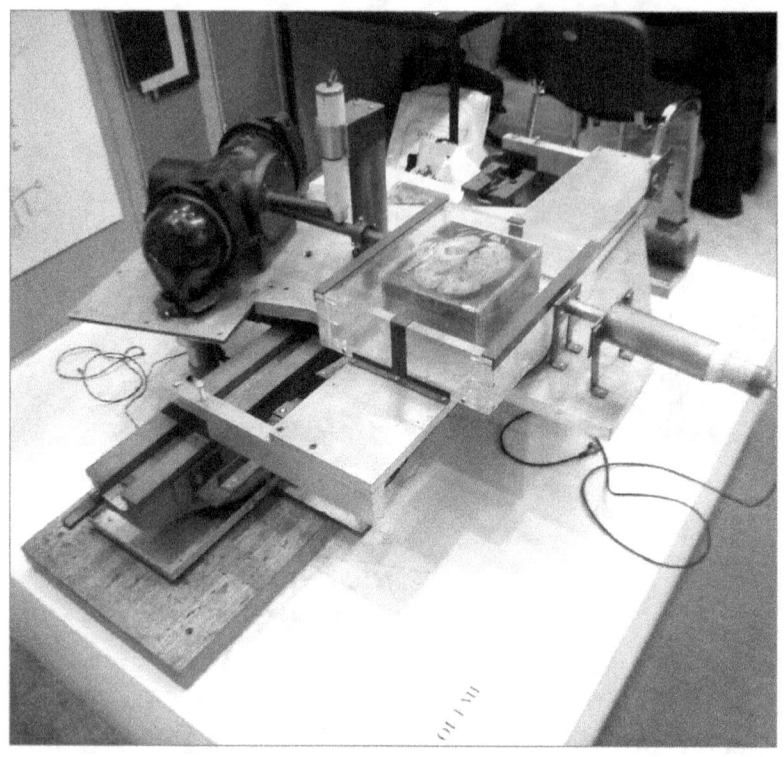

Hounsfield's prototype of the CT scanner built on the bed of the old lathe.

neurological images that Ambrose showed him with a dismissive "I can do better than that."

At the end of a seemingly unfruitful meeting Ambrose handed Hounsfield a jar, borrowed from the museum, containing a brain with a tumor and asked him for some proof of his invention. Five weeks later Hounsfield brought a picture of the brain, which showed the tumor and even areas of bleeding within the tumor. Ambrose was instantly stunned.

The Department of Health placed the order for a prototype and 3 clinical machines (£150 000 each) that would generate sufficient income to fund a fifth machine for Hounsfield and his team to keep and work on. The Department of Health would also fund half the remaining research costs (£69 000) and in exchange they would receive a small royalty on sales.

Thus Hounsfield assembled the team who assisted him with practical knowledge of radiology and provided tissue samples and test animals for scans. The team worked at Atkinson Morley's Hospital in Wimbledon which was chosen to avoid wide-spread publicity in the development phase.

This hospital was the busiest neurosurgical center in London. Neurosurgery there was led by W.McKissock who was concerned about the invasive character of neuroradiological examinations at that time and inspired the radiologists to look for alternative imaging techniques including ultrasound and nuclear medicine.

The development took place largely in secret. Frank Doyle supplied bone specimens, James Ambrose supplied brain specimens and Louis Kreel supplied abdominal specimens.

In 1968 Hounsfield was granted UK Patent No. 1,283,915 for "A Method of and Apparatus for Examination of a Body by Radiation such as X or Gamma Radiation".

Using gamma radiation Hounsfield successfully scanned an animal's brain in 1968. The scanning process took 9 days and required 2.5 hours to process the resulting 28,000 measurements on a high-speed computer. The scanning mechanism was then improved, faster data processing algorithms were developed, and advantage was taken of the rapid price-performance improvements of computers in the early 1970s.

A prototype EMI head scanner Mark I on October 1, 1971 provided the first clinical image of the female patient at Atkinson Morley's Hospital, Wimbledon. The equipment used a translate-rotate gantry and required a plastic cone or water bag for stabilization of the head. Each slice took 4 minutes and required 7 minutes for reconstruction. Post-processing took all night but produced a recognizable image of a brain tumor. Hounsfield exclaimed: "My God, it does work!" He and Ambrose both felt like footballers who had just scored the winning goal.

The skull was no longer a barrier to the radiological investigation of brain disorders making the discomfort of the pneumoencephalogram a thing of the past.

In 1979 Hounsfield was awarded the Nobel Prize for Physiology or Medicine shared with Allan M. Cormack. Neither of them had a degree in medicine or biology, or a doctorate in any field.

Hounsfield was appointed Commander of the

British Empire in 1976 and knighted in 1981.

He never married remaining a shy retiring bachelor, embarrassed by awards and honors. Hounsfield lived in modest surroundings, loved walking in the mountains, enjoyed music, played the piano by ear and retained his own time-clock wherever he was in the world, often seen wide awake in a hotel corridor in the early hours of the morning. Young people were happy getting his advice "not to worry about passing exams so long as you have understood the subject" and "not to worry about not getting up before 9 am!" He had no interest in power, position or possessions.

Sir Godfrey Newbold Hounsfield died on August 12, 2004 in Kingston upon Thames, England. ◆

Peter James Kerley

"He Who Made Time Made Plenty of It"

Kerley B lines are horizontal lines of striped shadows, usually best seen in the lower zones of the lungs. They are a sign of congestive heart disease and thought to be due to fluid in the interlobular septa.

Sir Peter James Kerley was born in Dundalk, Ireland, on October 27, 1900, the youngest of 13 children. Kerley was qualified at the National University in Dublin in 1923. He traveled to Vienna to study ear, nose, and throat diseases but changed his mind and dedicated a year for his radiological training. He obtained his medical degree from the University in Dublin in 1932.

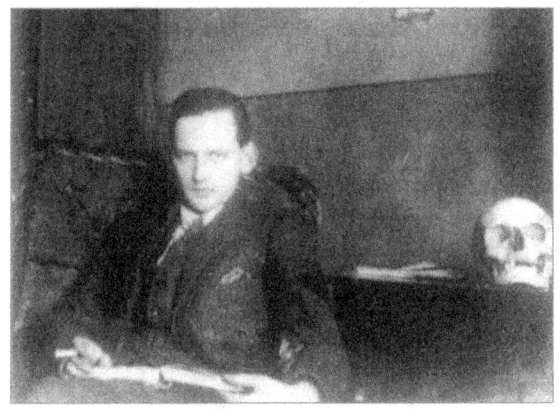

Sir Peter James Kerley*

Kerley was appointed Director of Radiology at the Westminster Hospital and National Heart Hospitals and became an adviser on radiology to the Ministry of Health. He was president of the radiology section of the Royal Society of Medicine in 1939-1940 and of

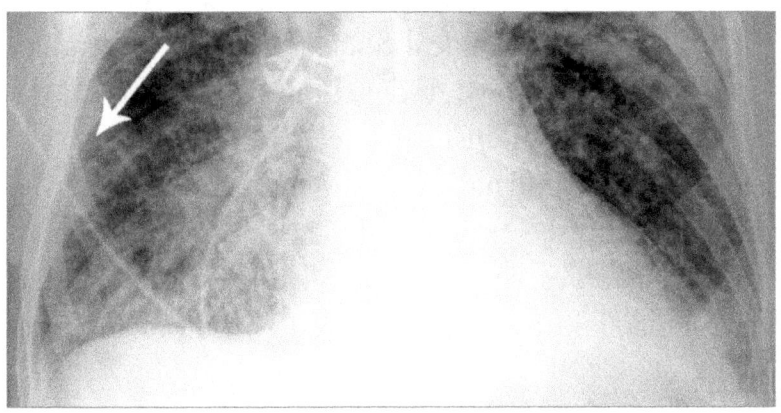

Kerley B lines - horizontal lines are a sign of congestive heart disease and are due to fluid in the interlobular septa.

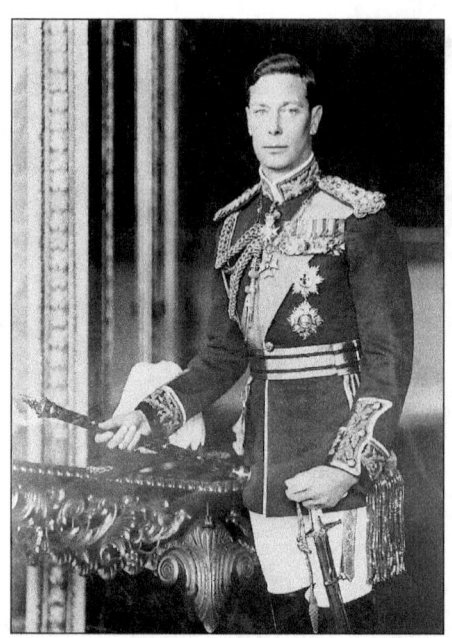

|| King George VI

the Faculty of Radiologists from 1952 to 1955. Kerley was a founding member of the College of Radiology, and later its president. He was an honorary member of the Chicago Radiological Society and the Australian College of Radiology, and Fellow of Honour of the Faculty of Radiologists in Ireland. He became the Editor of the Journal of Radiology, and later wrote the six volume "Textbook of x-ray diagnosis", which includes the description of the Kerley B lines of left ventricular failure, and the A & C lines on the chest X-ray.

In recognition of distinguished services to the Royal House he was made Commander of the Royal

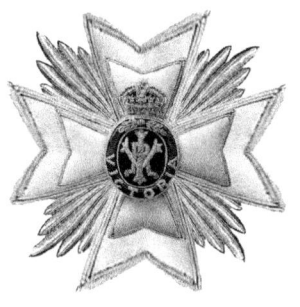Victorian Order in 1952 and Knight Commander of the Royal Victorian Order twenty years later.

He showed an Irish disregard for time, believing that "he who made time made plenty of it". He was a lover of wine and food, a superb fisherman and a good shot. On his trout fishing in Scotland, King George VI was among his companions. When the local doctor suggested an x-ray for the monarch, Kerley arranged the procedure back in London and broke the news of lung tumor to the King.

Sir Peter James Kerley died on March 15, 1979. The Sir Peter Kerley Lecture of the Royal College of Radiologists is named for him. ◆

Robert Kienböck

From Peaks of Glory
to the Depths of Depression

Kienböck's disease or Kienböck's malacia is an avascular necrosis of the lunate bone of the wrist. It was described by Austrian radiologist Robert Kienböck. He was born on January 11, 1871 in Vienna.

Graduating from Schottengymnasium, Robert Kienböck became one of the best students of his time in the medical school in Vienna. After getting his MD degree in 1895 he traveled to London and Paris where the news about the discovery of new rays reached him. There he also witnessed the first attempts of radiographic imaging. After his return to Vienna in 1897, Kienböck started working as an assistant to Leopold von Schrötter, internist and laryngologist. At

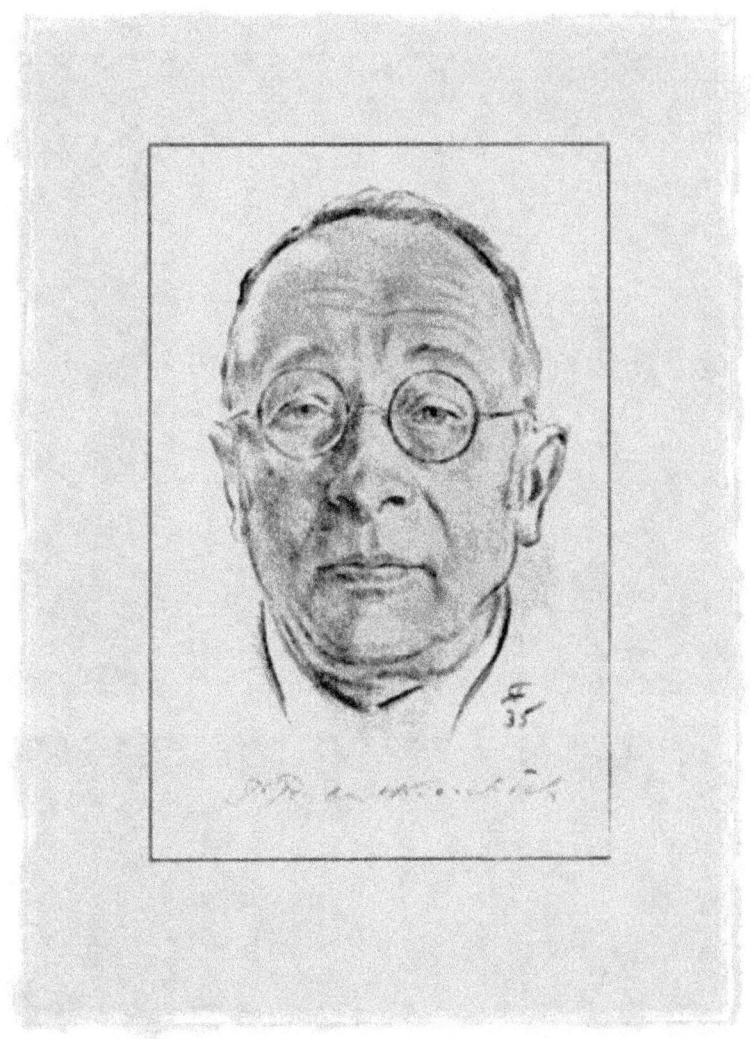

the same time he began to learn how to use the new rays. As was usual for him, he was very successful. Doctors from other hospitals started sending him the patients for diagnosis. Prospects for success were opening for this young and talented physician.

However, in 1899, like a bolt from the blue, the

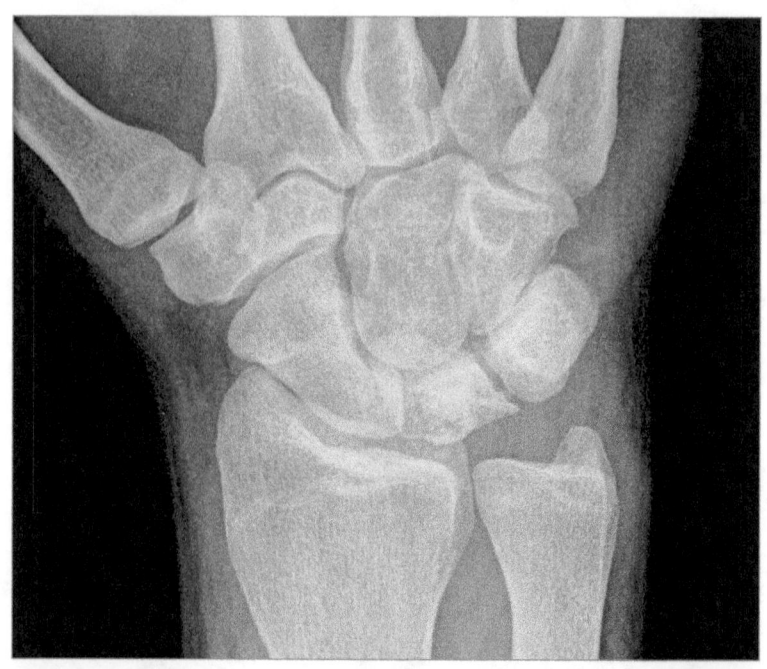

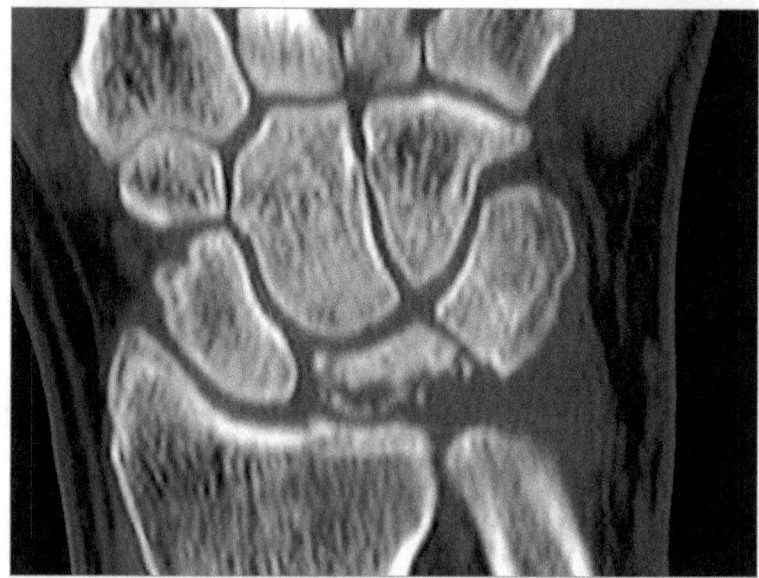

‖ *Kienböck malacia of the lunate bone.*

infamous gas bribery scandal in Vienna had erupted around his father, the famous and successful lawyer Karl Kienböck, making waves which seriously impeded Karl Kienböck. He was blamed for attempting to bribe the city council. Probably it is at this time that Kienböck – the father - realized that his son's decision not to follow his steps in law practice proved to be right.

Robert Kienböck was so successful in his x-ray activity that he managed to open his own private x-ray institute in the same year - 1899. With his friend and colleague, Leopold Freund, they fathered the new treatment method which would develop into radiotherapy. In 1905, Kienböck invented the Quantimeter to measure radiation dose which was received enthusiastically and helped in quantifying radiation exposure.

In 1910 Kienböck published his famous article on traumatic malacia of the lunate, providing the earliest description of avascular necrosis of the lunate bone. Although over the years Kienböck's proposed trauma-related etiology of the disease did not find support, it did not diminish the value of the article. The quality of the detailed description of the different phases of the malacia in the 1910 article was the result of years of effort spent by Kienböck in refining and perfecting the use of x-rays. This work represented an outstanding scientific achievement of that time.

That same year of 1910, at the climax of his scientific career, the almost fatal accident happened. A passionate and experienced rider, Kienböck fell from his horse. Immediately afterwards he was kicked by the horse and fell on the ground with severe open basal skull fracture. It was a medical miracle that he survived the trauma. After the long recovery it became apparent that people were meeting another Robert Kienböck. Not only the hearing impairment and nervous irritability were striking. A quiet, isolated closet scientist scholar emerged instead of the previously cheerful, outgoing sports lover.

He continued to publish works on bone and joint pathology including Paget disease and von Recklinghausen syndrome and was elected as the first president of the newly founded Austrian Radiology Society in 1934. However, the early Robert Kienböck was never to come again. In the early 1930s, Kienböck started working on a multivolume manuscript dedicated to diagnosis of bone and joint disease.

Austria's fall under control of the Nazi Third Reich in 1938 opened the darkest period in the history of Alma Mater Rudolphina (University of Vienna). 153 of 197 members of the medical faculty were fired almost immediately for being of Jewish origin, married to Jews or for being unwanted by the new regime for political reasons. Instead of 491 courses offered before the Anschluss, only 259 could be held after. The

CIVIC SCANDAL IN VIENNA.

ALLEGED GAS BRIBERY.

The text of a document has been published in Vienna purporting to he signed by Dr Leopold Teltscher on behalf of the Imperial Continental Gas Association, promising a commission of 60,000 florins, or £50,000, to Doctor Karl Kienboeck, a lawyer in Vienna, subject to payments of 100,000 florins to an assistant priest named Joseph Dittrich, and 75,000 florins to one Sigmund Freund, both of Vienna, provided that by their efforts, and especially by the intervention of Dittrich, a settlement was arranged between the Gas Association and the Vienna Town Council. In that event, the document says, the rest of the commission, after the deduction of the two sums specially mentioned, was to be paid either to Dr. Keinboeck alone, or to him and to other persons who contributed to or were interested in the settlement between the gas company and the town.

£50,000 FOR TOWN COUNCILLORS.

It has been asserted by a Vienna newspaper that the £50,000 was destined to bribe Town Councillors to vote for the

Article from Hawke's Bay Herald published on July 29, 1899 with the details of scandal involving Robert Kienböck's father.

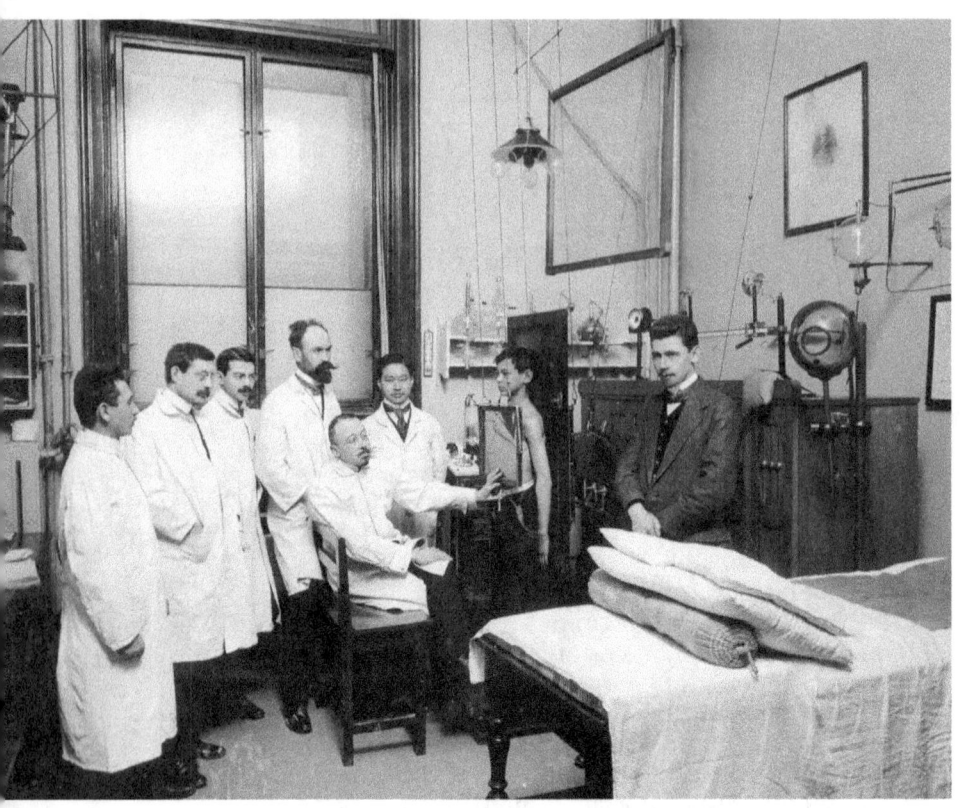

Examining the patient: Kienböck with junior physicians*

vacant posts were filled with persons mainly from the junior ranks of the faculty. The once leading medical school never recovered from this disaster. Neither did victims of the racial "cleansing". Kienböck's fellow professor and friend, Leopold Freund, was forced into exile and died impoverished in Belgium in 1943. Some of the expelled committed suicide or perished in concentration camps. The evicted and those who survived were discouraged from returning.

After publishing the eighth volume of his book in 1942, Kienböck suffered two strokes which caused a depression that grew more serious and made him unable to continue his scientific work. Although after the war he was elected honorary president of the Austrian Radiology Society, he would no longer write.

Robert Kienböck died in Vienna on September 7, 1953. At the age of 83, he was one of the last of the first generation of radiologists. Those who had had no teachers. Those who had to find for themselves the answers to all the questions. Those who had established the specialty and launched it into existence and progress. His life was not affected by the harmful effects of radiation exposure but personal and historical catastrophes deformed and changed it mercilessly. ◆

Emil Anthony Naclerio

Saving Martin Luther King

Naclerio V-sign is a V-shaped collection of air in the left lower mediastinum and along the diaphragm which is seen in pneumomediastinum. One limb of the V is produced by mediastinal air outlining the left lower lateral mediastinal border and the other limb is produced by air between the parietal pleura and medial left hemidiaphragm.

This sign was described in 1957 by surgeon Emil Anthony Naclerio. He was born in Brooklyn, New York on March 21, 1915. After graduation from Marquette Medical School in Wisconsin, Naclerio completed an advanced training in broncho-pulmonary surgery at Overholt Clinic in Boston. In 1950 he was recruited

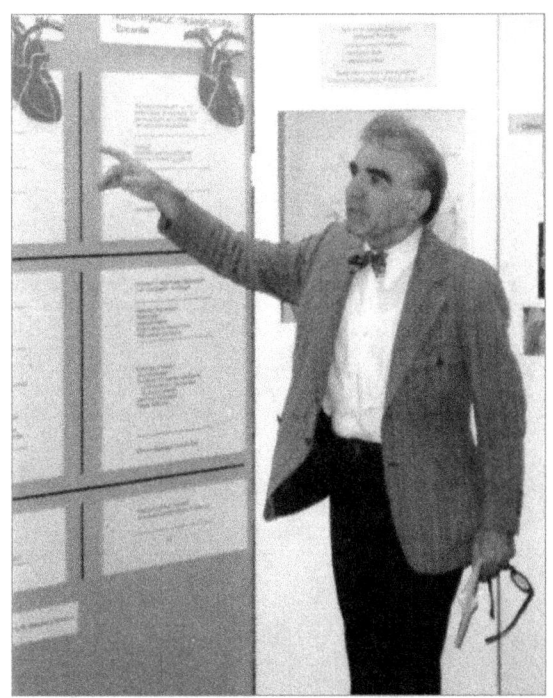

Emil Anthony Naclerio*

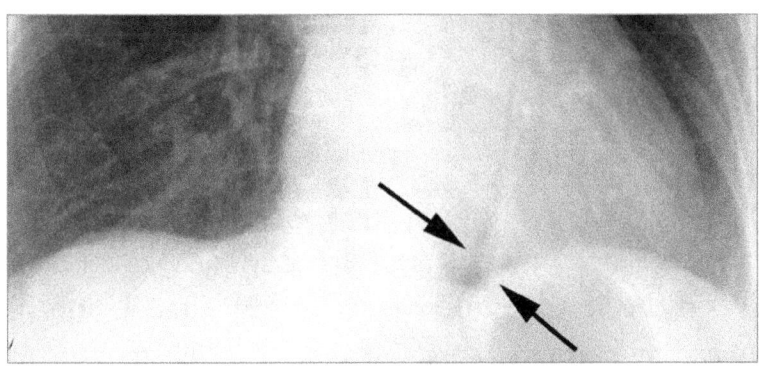

*Naclerio V-sign - V-shaped collection of air dissecting
along diaphragmatic and mediastinal fascial planes in
the region of the lower esophagus**

Martin Luther King, Jr.
Dexter Avenue Baptist Church
454 Dexter Avenue
Montgomery 4, Alabama

Amherst 3-3970

January 6, 1959

Dear Dr. Naclerio:

Ever since leaving New York I have been intending to write you at least a note to express my great appreciation to you for all that you did to preserve my life. Your skilled surgery, coupled with your genuine concern for me as a patient, combined to bring me from a very low ebb in my life to blooming health again. Please know that I will remember your gestures of goodwill so long as the cords of memory shall lengthen.

I hope you have received our gift by now. It is simply a little way to express our gratitude to you for all that you did to ease the load of a difficult period in our lives.

With best wishes to you and yours for health and happiness in 1959. I am

Sincerely yours,

Martin Luther King, Jr.

Dr. Emil Naclerio
35 East 35th Street
New York 16, New York

MLK:mlb

Letter written by M.L.King Jr. to Dr.E.Naclerio after convalescence

as a thoracic surgeon at Harlem Hospital. Upon his arrival at Harlem Hospital, Naclerio became known as an enthusiastic expert who broke the traditional "traffic rules" to reach the emergency cases which came in. In 1957 Naclerio published the article describing an early roentgen clue - the V sign in the diagnosis of spontaneous rupture of the esophagus. Despite the common practice in those days that the name of the department head was placed on a paper describing breakthrough research conducted in the department, the 1957 article by Naclerio was published under only his name.

On September 20, 1958, as the thoracic surgeon on call, Naclerio helped save the life of Martin Luther King Jr. after a stabbing by Izola Ware Curry. Stabbed with a 7-inch letter opener, King was taken to Harlem Hospital. Emil Naclerio, John Cordice and a chief resident, Leo Maitland, were the surgeons who removed the weapon from King's chest and operated on him for two-and-a-half hours. Photos of Emil Naclerio checking on King at the bedside were splashed across newspapers around the world. The operation and the involvement of the Department Chair, Aubre Maynard, would later be furnished sometimes with incorrect details and even many years after, would still spark controversies of the versions regarding the real events which took place in the operating room. These controversies would outlive the participants of the events.

Later in life, Naclerio helped to develop methods for inserting pacemakers and wrote books on chest injuries. Emil Naclerio died of congestive heart failure on October 14, 1985 in Brooklyn, New York. ◆

Edwards Albert Park

A Giant with a Gentle Touch

P ark's corner - metaphyseal corner fractures through the weakened lucent metaphyses.

Edwards Albert Park was born in Gloversville, New York on December 30, 1877. He died in Nova Scotia, Canada on July 11, 1969. Park was educated at Phillips Andover Academy and Yale. He earned his MD from Columbia's College of Physicians and Surgeons, in 1905. He went for a 6-month pediatric residency at the New York Foundling Hospital, with John Howland as an attending physician. In 1912, Howland, Professor of Pediatrics at Johns Hopkins, invited Park to work at Baltimore. There Park launched his research into rickets. With great thoroughness, Park went on to investigate the anatomy and biochemistry of normal and abnormal bone growth. This was a life-

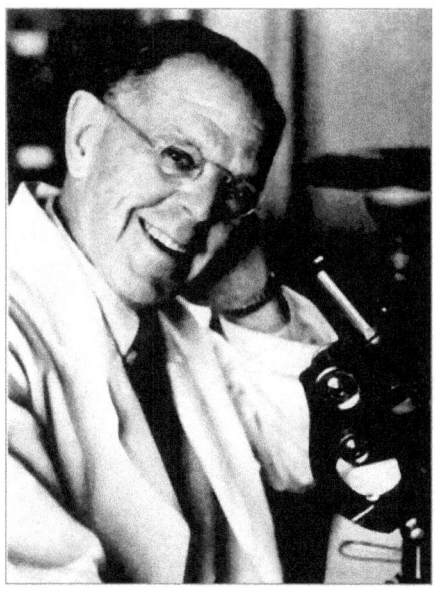

‖ *Edwards Albert Park**

long interest until his last scientific publication some 50 years later. Park married Ms. Agnes Bevan whom he had met in London. After returning from France where he was with the American Red Cross in World War I, Park accepted the Professorship of Pediatrics at Yale. Seven years later he came back to Johns Hopkins as Howland's successor and stayed at Johns Hopkins as Professor of Pediatrics and Pediatrician-in-Chief until his retirement in 1947.

Friends called him Ned and remembered him as a giant with a gentle touch, who left his mark on pediatrics and on many pediatricians. He was described as an ideal *chef de clinique*, providing an abundance of research problems for his doctors. He spared others

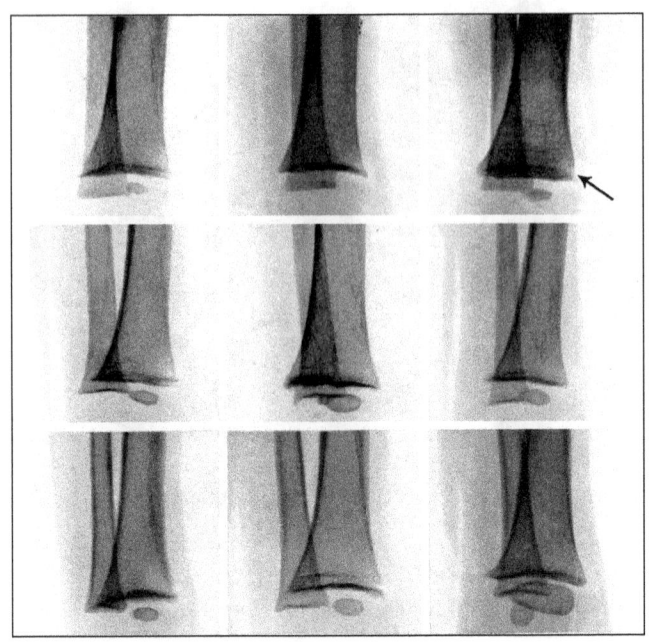

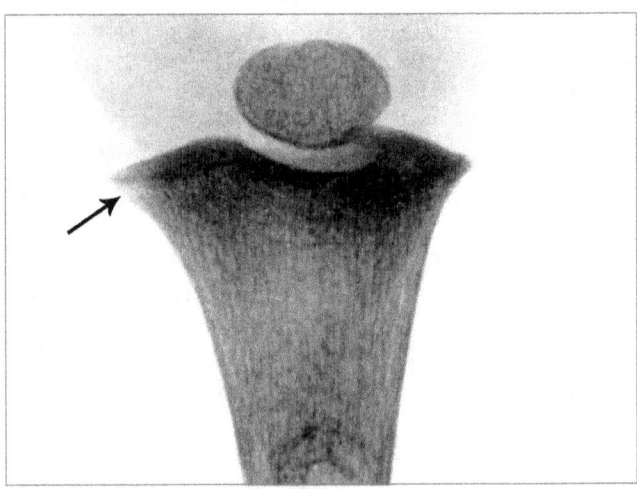

Park's corner - spot of rarefaction at the metaphyseal corner of the bone in scurvy*

from his criticism carrying self-criticism to an almost masochistic pitch. Park had a real gift of appreciation. It was said that "all Ned's geese are swans."

For more than thirty years summers were spent in Northeast Margaree, Nova Scotia, Canada. He built a cabin there and spent time fishing, physical exercise and the simple life. His mind remained clear until the end. He died in Margaree, in the place he loved.

Park was appreciated for his teaching which built foundations for pediatrics, establishing the nation's first pediatric sub-specialty clinics in pediatric cardiology, tuberculosis, endocrinology, seizure disorders and child psychiatry.

As a scientist he is credited with the discovery of Vitamin D in preventing rickets.

Interestingly, having contributed to the study of rickets, the radiological sign named after him was described in a publication on scurvy in 1935. Reading Park's articles describing the x-ray findings in scurvy, one understands how the experience and knowledge he gained studying rickets helped him to analyze changes in scurvy. In Park's original articles the spots of rarefaction at the corners of the bone appear in the x-ray, corresponding to pathologic findings of the thinned or disappearing cortex. "The cortex always showed fracture, and about the points of fracture the rarefaction processes seemed to be in full operation". ◆

Karl Francis Pelkan

"This is the Kind of Man We Want in This Country"

Metaphyseal beaks, associated with marginal fractures are known as Pelkan spurs and are seen in scurvy.

Karl Francis Pelkan was born August 16, 1890 in Marburg, Styria, Austria. His original name was Karl Pelikan. He was one of six children of a small candy factory owner. At the age of 16 he left the home and worked on different jobs to collect money for the trip to America. Accompanied by his cousin and having $25 with him, he came to Ellis Island on board the IMS *Kronprinzessin Cecilie* on August 3,

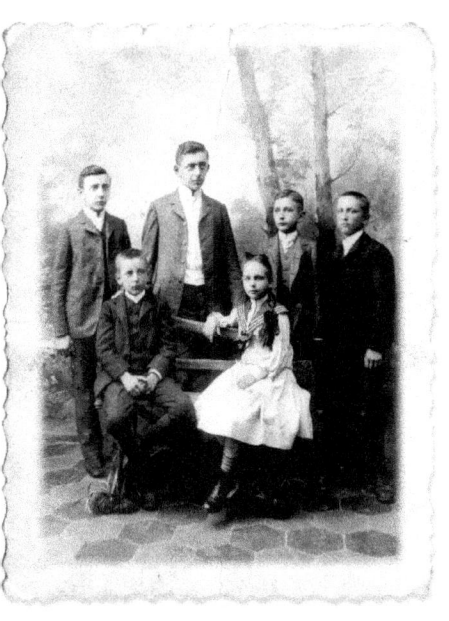

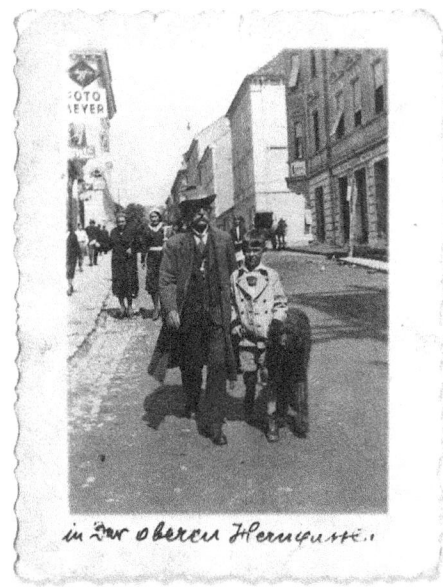

in der oberen Herrngasse.

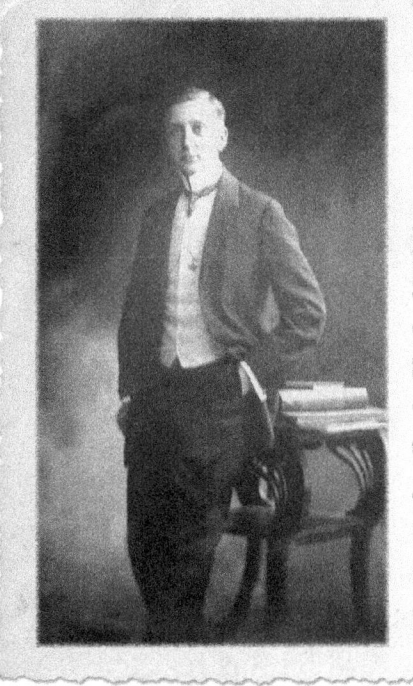

Previously unpublished
photographs from the family
archives. Karl Pelikan with his
siblings (upper left) and his
father (upper right).
Young Karl Pelikan.
Courtesy of Jennifer
McCaffrey, granddaughter of
Dr.Pelkan

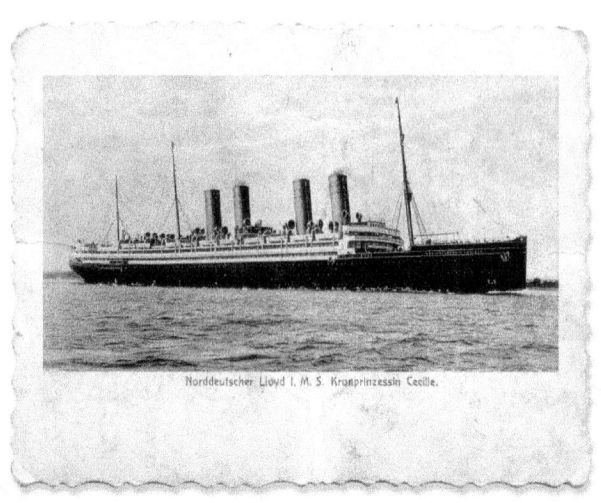

Norddeutscher Lloyd I. M. S. Kronprinzessin Cecilie.

| *IMS Kronprinzessin Cecilie as it looked*
| *at the time when Karl Pelikan traveled*
| *on board on his way to America.*

1909. After immigration he moved from one job to another, sometimes almost penniless. Once, working as a sign painter he had to escape his angry boss on the streetcar, leaving his coat and hat behind and being afraid to go back and pick them up. Being too poor to buy heavy clothes for cold winter in Chicago, he moved to warmer California.

Based on the evidence of his granddaughter, Ms. Jennifer McCaffrey, Karl dropped "i" from his surname while coming through Ellis Island. However, he kept signing himself as "Karl Pelikan" on his World War I draft record and, in 1923, while applying for the passport needed for the journey to Germany. On his WWI draft card he was registered

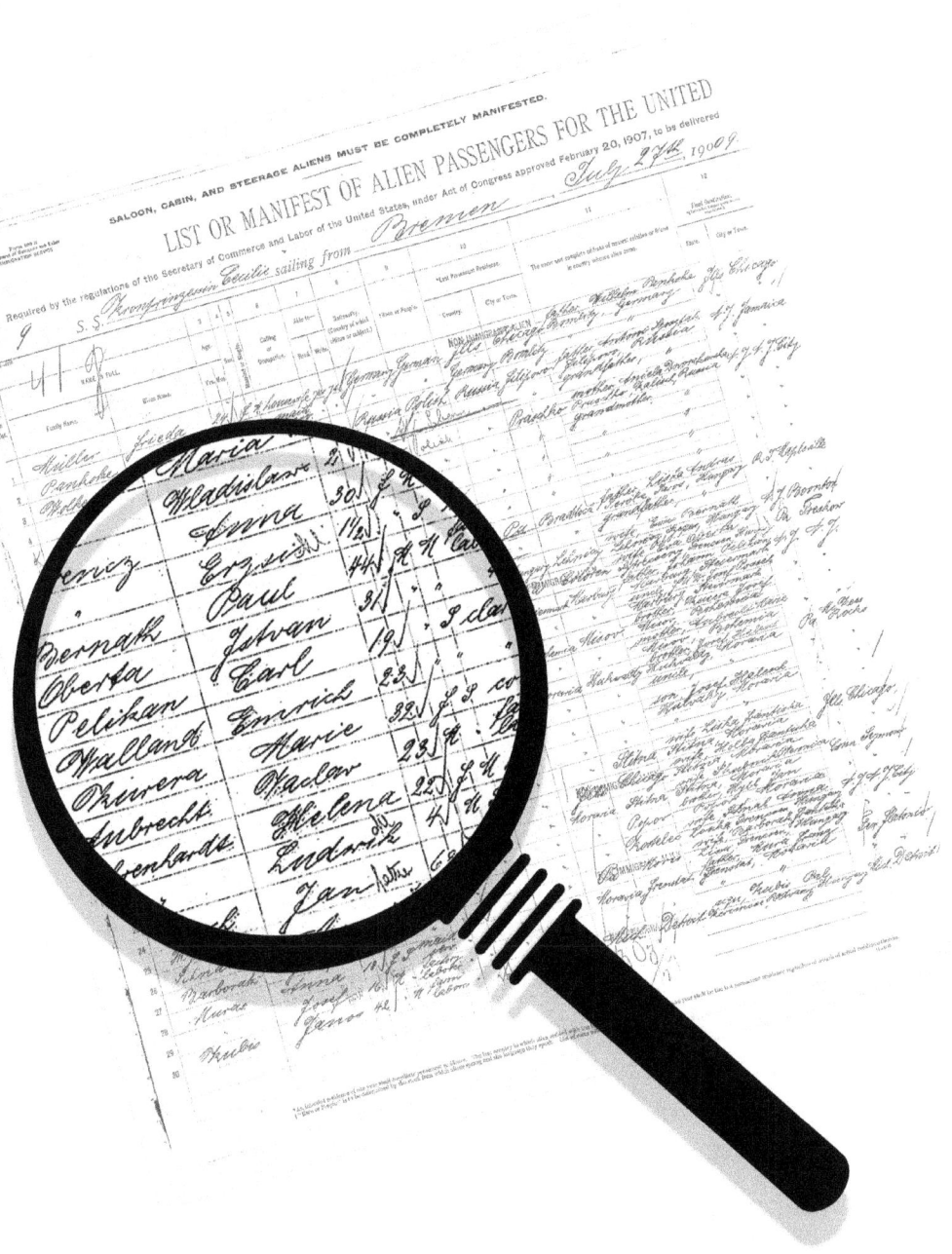

*List of passengers of Kronprinzessin Cecilie from
July 27, 1909 with the name of Pelikan Carl**

|| *K.Pelkan's Cum Laude MD Diploma from Harvard University.*

as a medical student at the University of California, answering "No" to the question whether married or single. He was exempted from service after physical exam. He was naturalized at Superior Court, San Francisco, California on December 1, 1916. When he was asked: "What kind of country is America?", he answered in broken English: "It is a country where people elect their representatives and make their own laws". The judge declared: "This is the kind of man we want in this country".

After pre-med courses at the University of

California, Berkeley, he entered Harvard University and earned his medical degree cum laude in 1923. After more study in Europe, he returned to San Francisco as an assistant professor of pediatrics at the medical school of the University of California. He opened a practice in San Jose in 1926 and married May Ring in 1927. His colleagues remembered him as remarkably dedicated to his work and his patients, working on Sundays and having the phone line connected directly to his home. In the years of the Depression he treated patients who often could not pay. They would bring boxes with fruits and vegetables instead making Mrs.Pelkan fill the basement with preserves. He was chief of pediatrics at O'Connor Hospital and taught at the nursing school. People remembered him "as my pediatrician and my mother's". In retirement he and his wife traveled extensively. Coming back, they sold their San Jose home and moved to a retirement

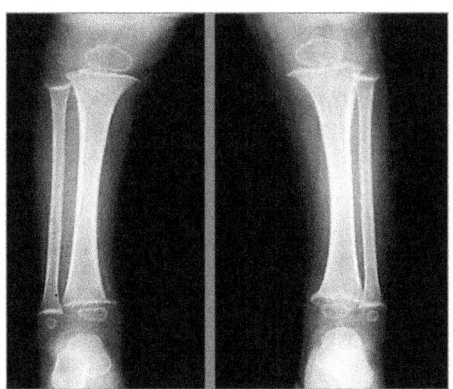

Pelkan spurs - metaphyseal marginal fracture in infantile scurvy*

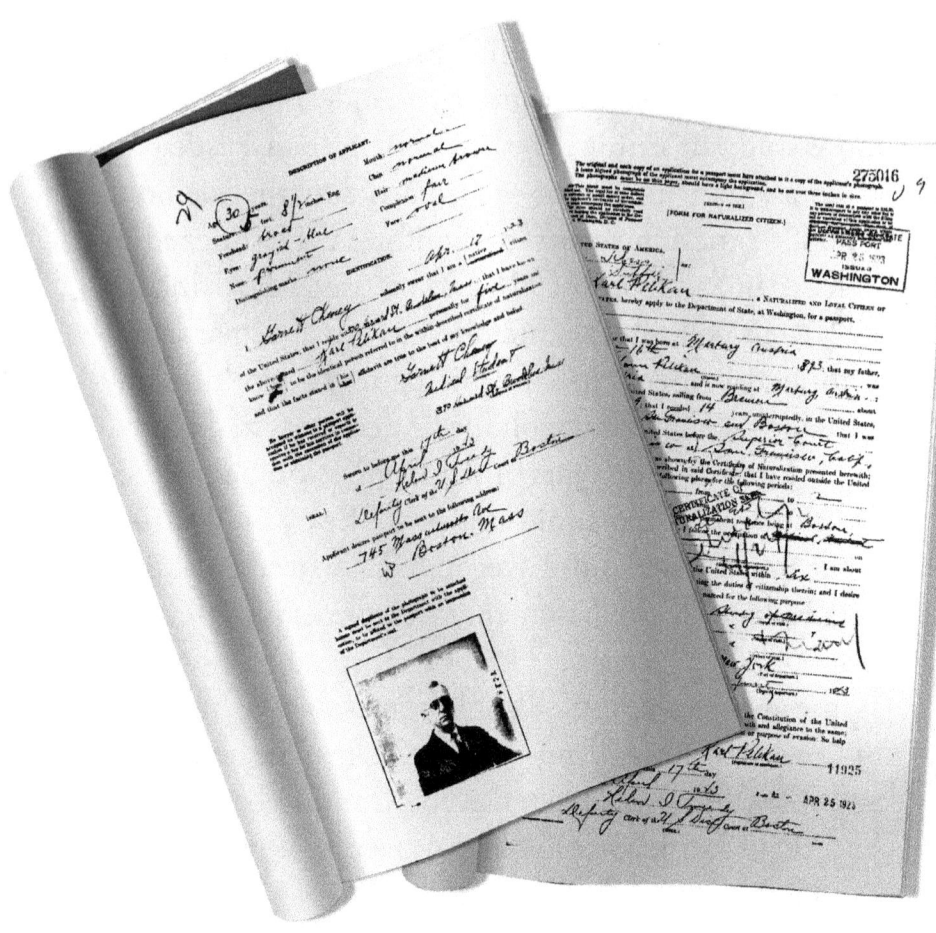

Passport application. It was signed in 1923 as "Karl Pelikan" despite dropping "i" from the surname many years before*

complex in San Francisco.

Working for the George Williams Hooper Foundation for Medical Research, University of California, San Francisco, Pelkan published three articles on the physiology of the phenols in the Journal of Biological Chemistry.

In 1925 he worked at the Department of Pediatrics, Harvard Medical School, and the Children's and Infant's Hospitals, Boston. There, Pelkan published "The roentgenogram in early scurvy". He was the third (after E. Fraenkel and H. Wimberger) to investigate the diagnosis of early scurvy, particularly borderline cases, based on roentgenograms from cases of scurvy in human beings and on the findings of experimental scurvy in the guinea-pig. Interestingly, it is only in the text of the article that he described "a small spur at the lateral edge of the epiphyseal line" and wrote: "Clinically, the cases which show the lateral spur are usually far advanced, with tremendously swollen and painful extremities and all the usual symptoms of scurvy. The lateral spur of the epiphyseal line is evidence of a full-blown, advanced case". Because it had no value for the diagnosis of early cases, "before any of the accepted clinical symptoms have appeared", the description of the spurs, which were later given his name by citing authors, did not find its place in the conclusions. Pelkan's scope of interests and expertise was very wide and included clinical work, pathology, roentgenology, biochemistry and experimental medicine.

101 years old, Karl Pelkan died April 17, 1992 of cancer in the retirement complex in San Francisco, CA. People burst in tears, learning of his death. ◆

Leo George Rigler

Pneumoperitoneum and 200 articles

R igler sign is the double-wall sign of free intraperitoneal air. Leo George Rigler was born October 16, 1896, in Minneapolis, Minnesota. Rigler received his MD degree in 1920 at the University of Minnesota. Following a 1-year internship in the St. Louis City Hospital, he shortly worked as a general practitioner in New England, North Dakota. He returned to the University of Minnesota to take a 1-year position as a teaching fellow in the department of internal medicine. In 1923–1926 he worked as a radiologist at the Minneapolis General Hospital. During this period he learned radiology at the

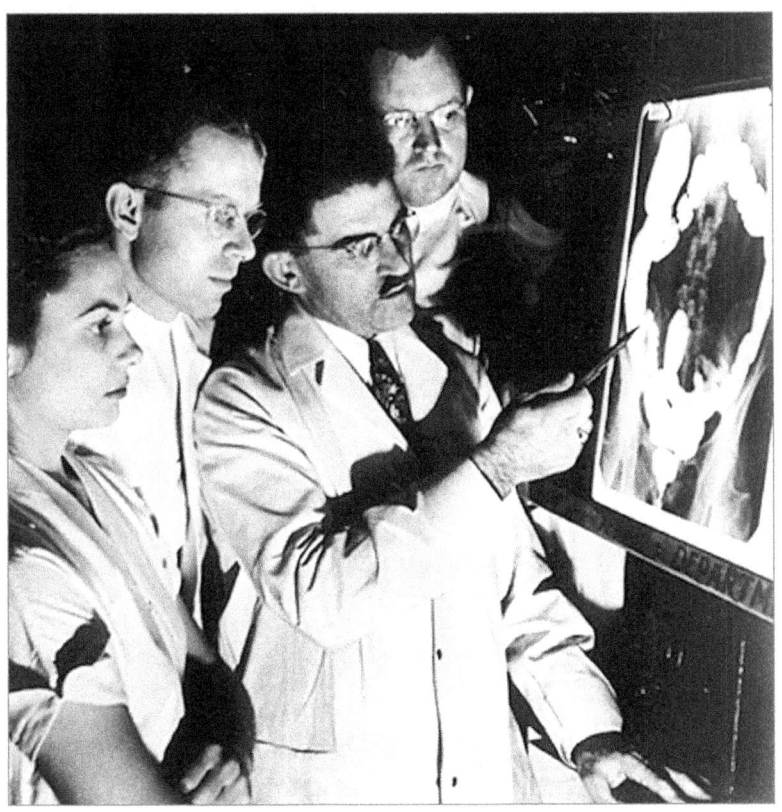

|| *Leo George Rigler**

Battle Creek Sanatorium from J. T. Case and at the University of Michigan from P. J. Hickey. Rigler also worked as an assistant in anatomy at the University of Minnesota and was engaged in the private practice of radiology.

In 1924, with $1000 funding from D. Lyon, the dean of the University of Minnesota Medical School, Rigler left for Europe to visit various clinics but primarily he spent a year in Stockholm at the

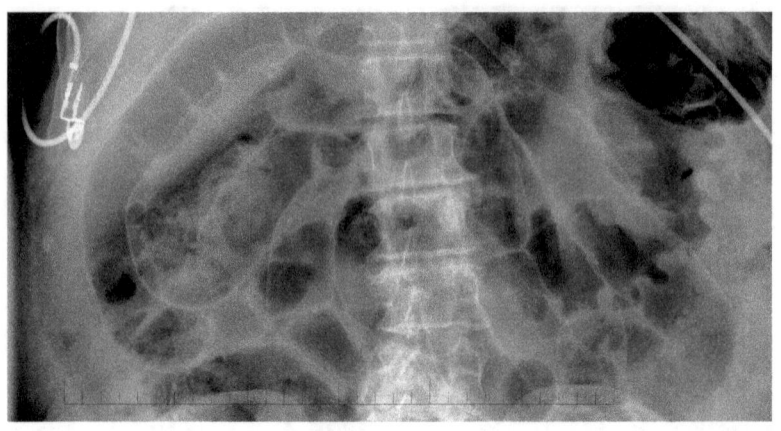

Rigler sign – air outlines the bowel wall from both sides in pneumoperitoneum.

Karolinska Institute where he was Dr. Gosta Forssell's first American trainee. Studying there, he learned to speak Swedish.

On his return from Europe, being 31 years old, Rigler got a full-time appointment as an associate professor of radiology at the University of Minnesota. This was the first such appointment ever at that university. Two years later, he became a full professor. In 1933 at the age of 37 years, he became chair of the department of radiology - the first full-time chairman of radiology at the University of Minnesota. He held that position until 1957. After the American Board of Radiology was incorporated and organized at a meeting in May 1934, Rigler was certified by the American Board of Radiology in 1934 while a full professor. He was the 68th candidate to receive this recognition. In 1957 Rigler moved to the West Coast, where he worked as the executive director of the Cedars of Lebanon–Mount Sinai Hospitals. In 1963 he returned to academic medicine getting the appointment of a professor of radiology at the University of California, Los Angeles (UCLA). At UCLA, he directed the postgraduate program in diagnostic radiology. He held this position until his death in 1979 at age 83.

Rigler occupied a host of prestigious positions in medicine. He was consultant to the Armed Forces Institute of Pathology and the United States Public Health Service and a member of the National Cancer Advisory Council, the Committee on Academic Radiology of the National Academy of Sciences, the Committee on Radiology of the National Research Council, and the Medical Advisory Board of the Tel Aviv University Medical School.

Among his honors and awards were the gold medals of the Radiological Society of North America as well as of the American College of Radiology, the Crookshank Medal from the British Faculty of Radiologists, an honorary fellowship from the Royal College of Radiology, and the Caldwell Medal from the American Roentgen Ray Society.

Rigler held many official posts in medical organizations. He was president of the Radiological Society of North America (being the first Jew to take this position), the Fleischner Society, the Minnesota Radiological Society, and the Minnesota Pathological Society. He was also a chancellor of the American College of Radiology. Many awards and honors have been summarized in tributes to him. Rigler Lectureships were established during his lifetime, two in the United States and one in Israel. Leo Rigler was author or co-author of four books and over 200 articles.

In 1941, Rigler described four cases with a new sign with which the presence of free air in the peritoneal cavity could be recognized. Pneumoperitoneum made it possible to see the wall of gas-containing viscera on supine radiographs of the abdomen. In his report, Rigler emphasized that this sign was observed only when large quantities of free gas were present in the abdomen and that it frequently was observed in very ill patients in whom only limited radiographs of the abdomen could be obtained.

Leo George Rigler died on October 25, 1979 in Los Angeles, California. ◆

FATE OF THE PIONEERS

In 1905, after 10 years of exposure to X-rays, Dr G. Pirie began to experience "trouble" in his hands.

He wrote: "The skin cracked open, and it amused my comrades to see going about with sticking plaster all over them. Sometimes I would waken at night and find them tingling like fire. I was urged to give up the X-ray work and merely superintend, but I could never bring myself to cause others to take a risk that I would not take myself. I was told that nothing could be done. I like to draw a veil over these days."

He started using mustard oil and lead-lined goggles. Tumors developed on the right thumb and the fifth finger of his right hand. This required amputation and eventually he lost both his hands.

His eyesight also began to fail. He lost one eye and most of the sight from the other.

In 1926, when he was no longer able to continue working, he was awarded a Civil List pension and a Carnegie Hero Trust medal and pension. Dundee citizens presented him £1120 raised by subscription, in grateful recognition of his devoted service.

Richard Schatzki

"You Still Have to Work for It"

Schatzki ring – the lower esophageal ring structure was described by Richard Schatzki. He was born on February 22, 1901, in Clafeld, Germany. He was a son of Ferdinand Schatzki (1857-1910), an engineer from Bialystok (then Russian Empire) and Beate (née Stern) from Schmallenberg, Germany.

Richard Schatzki entered medical school when he was 19 years old. He studied at a number of medical schools including Munich, Frankfurt, Freiburg, and Tübingen and graduated from the University of Berlin in 1925. He got his MD after internships on the medical service at the West End Hospital in Berlin and the surgical service of the University Hospital in Frankfurt am Main. His original thinking was apparent when in the discussion of his MD

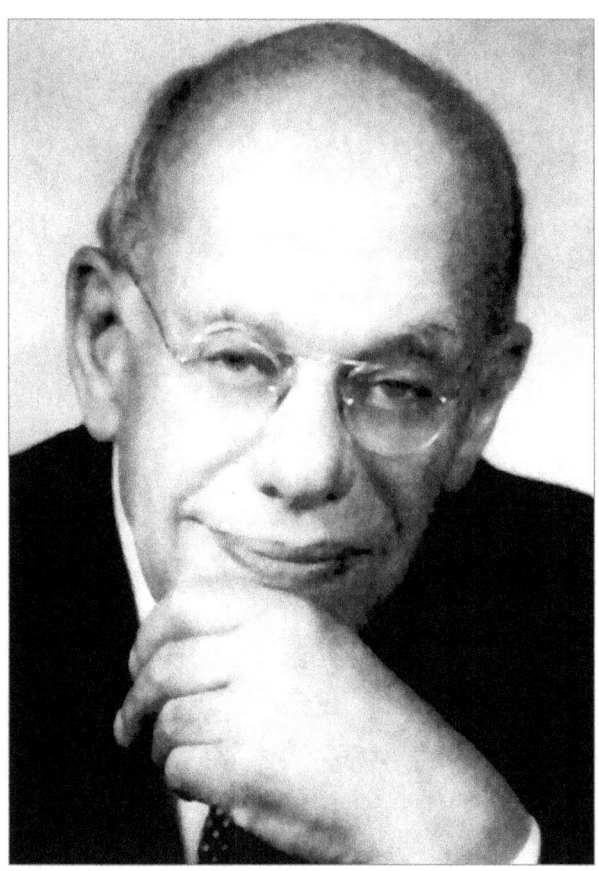

|| *Richard Schatzki**

thesis, Schatzki questioned the relationship between dermatomyositis, polymyositis, and scleroderma. Unfortunately, his professor crossed out this part of the discussion before publication of the thesis.

Schatzki spent 1926-1929 at the University Hospital in Frankfurt am Main. Believing that knowledge of radiology would help him in his career, he spent 15 months learning from Hans Heinrich

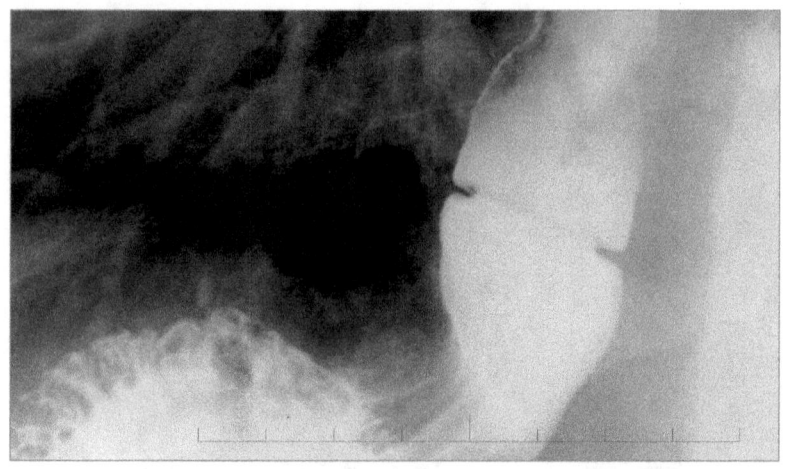

|| Schatzki ring in lower esophagus.

Berg who was the head of the radiology department of the medical clinic at Frankfurt and was the leading diagnostic radiologist in Germany at that time. In 1929, on Berg's recommendation, Schatzki became chief of the radiology department in the medical clinic at the University Hospital in Leipzig. In 1930 he married a physician, Margarete (Greta) Stern (1899-1981).

In Leipzig, Schatzki published the first of his numerous articles. His interest in gastro-intestinal radiology focused on esophageal and gastric varices, erosive gastritis and importance of relief studies of the gastrointestinal tract. He also published articles with one of the first descriptions of the radiographic findings in coarctation of the aorta and calcification of the adrenal gland in tuberculosis.

In 1933, as the Nazis rose to power, life became increasingly dangerous for the Schatzki family as for all other Jews in Germany. Richard's brother Erich, an internationally known aircraft designer and engineer who helped develop the German aircraft industry working for Junkers and budding Lufthansa airline as a test and then commercial pilot, had to flee to Holland. Faced with the danger of Nazi occupation he had to flee further to the USA where he helped design the famous P-47 Thunderbolt fighter plane, which bombed Germany. In late 1940s he moved to Israel to be one of the founders of the Israel Aircraft Industries. Another brother, Dr.Paul Schatzki, fled to Italy, served as a ship's surgeon in British Merchant Marine, was interned in Britain and sent on board HNT *Dunera* with 3000 intellectuals from Germany, half of them Jews, on the nightmare trip to Australia.

In 1933, Richard Schatzki's Dozent thesis was rejected on "racial grounds" according to newly enforced racial laws in Nazi Germany. As a consequence, Schatzki left Germany arriving with his wife and son Stefan (a future radiologist himself) in New York on July 26, 1933 on board the ship "*Bremen*". Records of his arrival indicated that he was going to his friend Dr. Alice Ettinger and that he had an inguinal hernia on the right side. He did not have any immediate prospect of employment when he immigrated to the

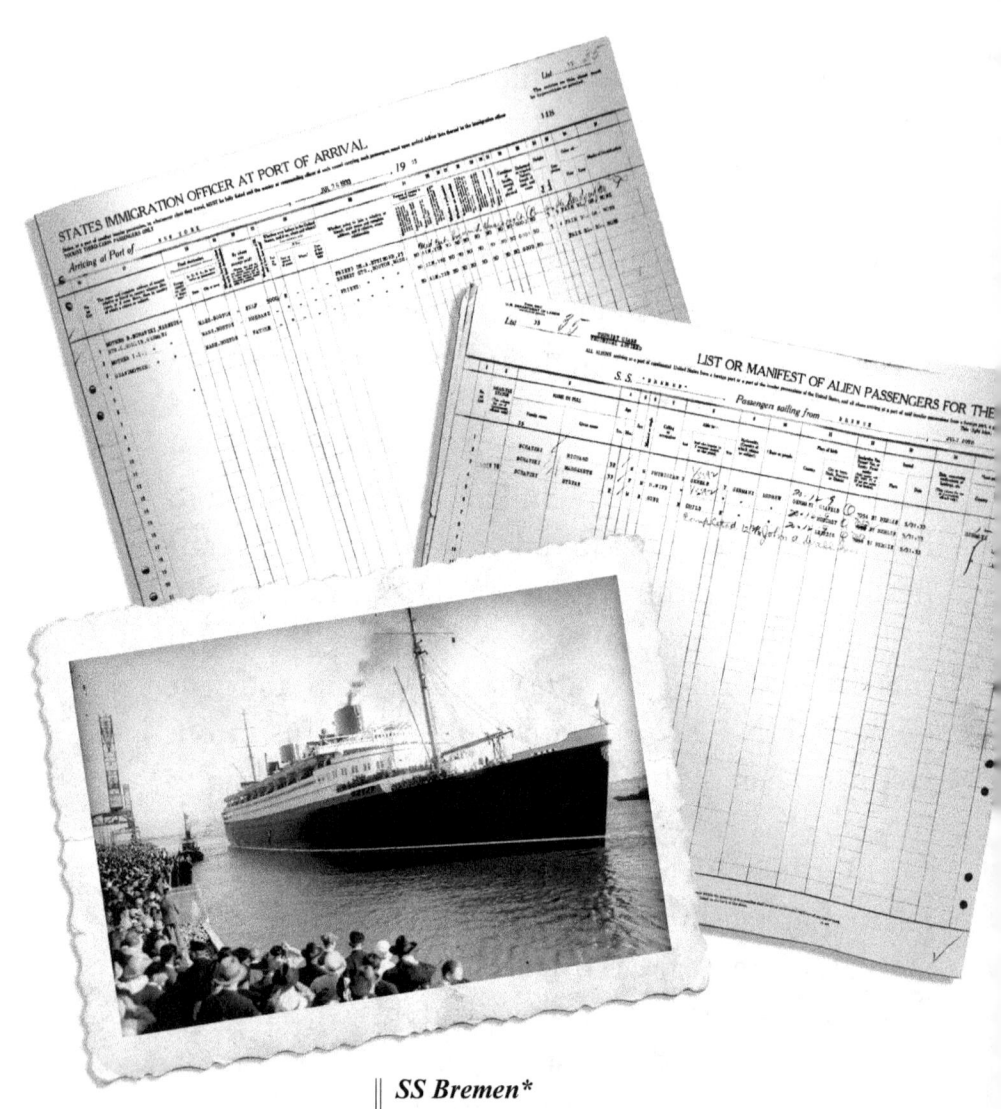

SS Bremen*

*List of passengers who arrived on July 20,
1933 on board of SS Bremen in New York:
Richard, Margaret and Stefan Schatzki.
They planned to stay with A.Ettinger in Boston**

United States. At the suggestion of Ettinger, another of Berg's students, he went to Massachusetts General Hospital (MGH), where one week later he gave a lecture on the demonstration of mucosal patterns in the esophagus, using relief studies of the esophagus. He presented in English and, as was common in the German tradition, without notes. Shortly afterward, he was offered a nonpaying position as an assistant in the radiology department. He lived on a small stipend from a committee formed to aid displaced scholars until 1935, when a paid position became available.

Richard Schatzki contributed to the process when in important ways, American radiology of those years was a specialty imported from Germany. The expertise and sometimes the equipment of German and Austrian refugee radiologists made Boston an early national leader in the field. There was little formal teaching in the radiology department in those years and most instruction resulted from the interactions between him and the residents while he interpreted films.

During World War II, Schatzki, feeling a deep debt to the United States, devoted a lot of effort to convince the Army to accept him. He served on active duty from June 1943 to April 1946 and reached the rank of lieutenant colonel, spending most of this time as a chief of radiology services at McGuire Hospital in Richmond, VA.

After World War II, Schatzki left MGH to become chief of the Radiology Department at the Mount Auburn Hospital in Cambridge, MA. He stayed in that position until 1967 and continued to work there until the age of 82 helping to transform Mount Auburn from an unsophisticated community hospital into one of the Harvard teaching hospitals with a modern radiology department and its own residency program. In 1984 the radiology department was named the "Richard Schatzki Department of Radiology".

In a series of articles between 1953 and 1963, together with John E. Gary, Schatzki described and defined the important entity, which is now generally known as the "Schatzki ring" - the lower esophageal ring structure. Schatzki himself believed that the recognition of the lower esophageal ring is perhaps his most important contribution to radiology.

Schatzki always emphasized the "art" of fluoroscopy and proper fluoroscopic technique for successful gastrointestinal fluoroscopy. Some of his philosophy about fluoroscopy was stated in a 1966 editorial discussing the impact of screen intensification. The title of the editorial was "You still have to work for it."

Schatzki was an associate clinical professor of radiology at Harvard Medical School and president of the New England Roentgen Ray Society. He was a member of most of the national and local radiology societies, a vice president of the American Roentgen Ray Society and an honorary member of the radiology societies of Brazil and Colombia. In 1973, Schatzki was awarded the Walter B. Cannon Medal from the Society of Gastrointestinal Radiologists.

On September 28, 1981 it was reported that when Richard Schatzki, then 79 years old, was behind the wheel and searching for his hearing aid, backed his 1979 Oldsmobile, the car rolled out the couple's driveway and hit 81-year-old Greta Schatzki. Mrs. Schatzki initially was either hit by the car or slipped on her way around the vehicle. She was taken to Mt. Auburn Hospital in Cambridge, to the place where the radiology department would carry the name of Richard Schatzki. She was pronounced dead. Richard Schatzki was treated for shock. Richard and Greta Schatzki had two sons – Stefan, a radiologist and George, Professor of Law.

Schatzki had many outside interests. He played the piano as good as a concert artist and often responded to requests for public performances. An effective way to get Richard Schatzki to speak out of town was to arrange an excellent quartet or trio.

Richard Schatzki died on January 19, 1992 in Lexington, Massachusetts. ◆

Alfred Baker Spalding

Gynecologist with Only One Article Dedicated to X-ray Findings

Spalding sign was described as an overlapping of the fetal skull bones on x-ray as a mark of intra-uterine fetal death.

Alfred Baker Spalding was born on July 19, 1874 in Atchison, Kansas.

He graduated with a bachelor degree from Stanford University in 1896. While at university he was on Walter Camp's first all American football team in 1895. He got his MD degree from Columbia University in 1900. Spalding worked as a surgeon at General Memorial Hospital, New York, then at Sloane Maternity Hospital in 1901-1902. He started

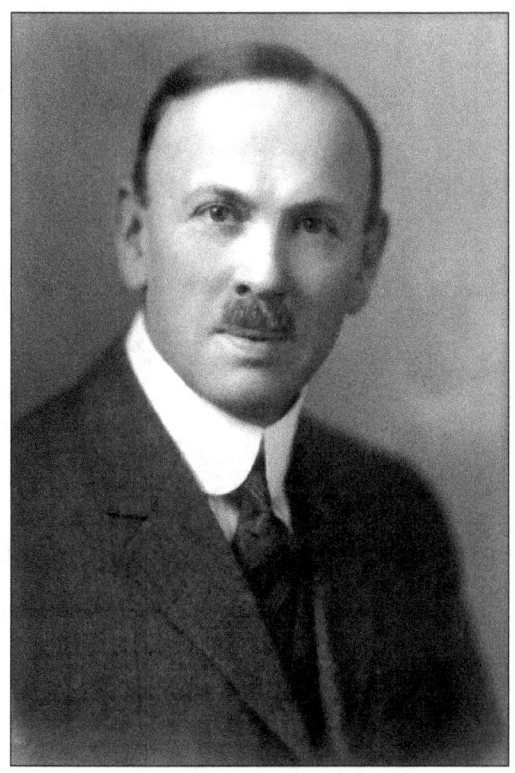

Alfred Baker Spalding*

working as an instructor in obstetrics and later became Professor of Obstetrics and Gynecology at University of California in 1902-1912. Spalding organized the San Francisco Maternity Hospital on January 1, 1904. In 1912 he was appointed Professor of Obstetrics and Gynecology at Stanford University and worked there until his retirement in 1930.

Spalding published articles on carcinoma of

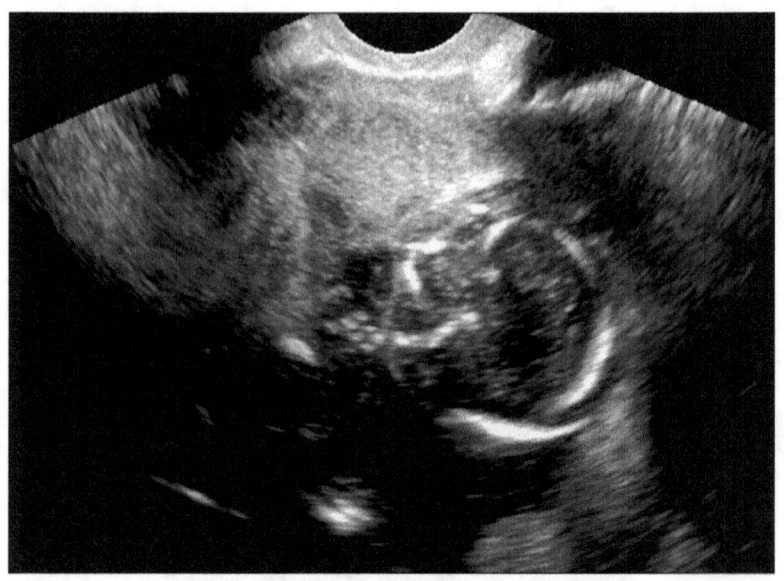

Spalding sign on ultrasound – overlapping cranial bones in fetal demise*

the uterus, venereal disease in patients suffering with sterility, prolapse of the uterus, eclampsia, hypertrophic pyloric stenosis, cesarian section, and the management of placenta previa. However, his only work dedicated to x-ray findings was published in 1922. Spalding presented a series which included three cases of intra-uterine death due to congenital syphilis which demonstrated the radiological sign that today is known by his name. It was later demonstrated that conditions sometimes produce a radiological appearance of overlap in a living fetus (false Spalding's sign). With the advance of obstetric sonography, the Spalding sign got recognition on ultrasound. Searching literature regarding Spalding sign reveals that this eponym was sometimes recorded as possessive (Spalding's sign) or with elimination of the possessive (Spalding sign).

Alfred Spalding died on November 27, 1942 in San Francisco, California. ◆

Eduard Stierlin

"Reliable to the Very End"
Famous Name in Psychiatry
Talented Surgeon
Unknown Titan

Stierlin sign, associated with tuberculous involvement of the ileocecum when terminal ileum empties directly into stenotic ascending colon with non-opacification of the fibrotic and contracted cecum, is well known in medical practices in areas where tuberculosis is common. However, the identity of the person who described this sign was quite obscure until recently. Scattered details and facts, assembled together created the image of the talented and brave physician, who distinguished himself in many fields and deserved respect and love of famous and honored superiors and colleagues.

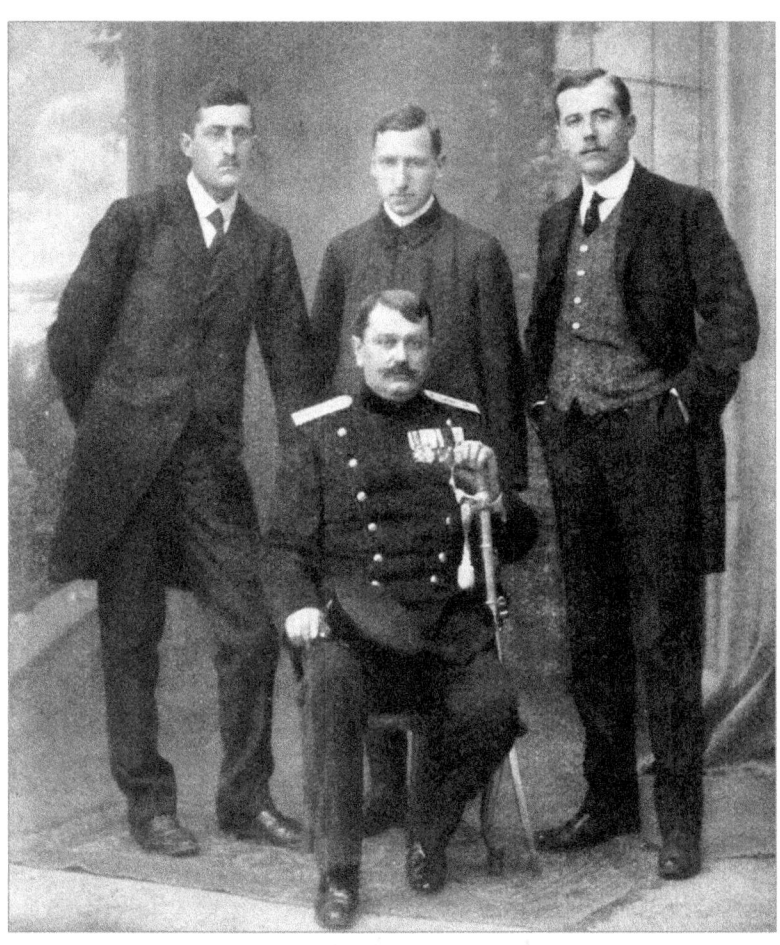

Eduard Stierlin (standing in the center) with other Basel surgeons Christoph Socin (left), Adolf Vischer (right) and B.Subotitsch (sitting), secretary of the Serbian Red Cross.

Eduard Stierlin was born in Zurich, Switzerland on February 3, 1878, son of Eduard Joseph (1839-1894), the chief engineer for Escher, Wyss and Co and Nannette (née Vögeli) (1855-1945) Stierlin. His father died when Eduard was 16 years old. Thanks to the efforts of his devoted mother, the childhood of Eduard and his 4 siblings in Zurich was sunny and carefree. After successfully passing his high school exam in Zurich, he became a machinist working for the same company as his father, dreaming of a career as engineer. However, he had to give this up since physically he was not suited for it.

Stierlin studied medicine in Zurich, Berlin, Hamburg, and Tübingen getting his MD in 1903. He passed his state exam in Bern in 1907.

Stierlin traveled to France, Germany, Belgium, South America and Italy. To Valparaiso he went as the ship's doctor. In 1909 Stierlin published his first work named "Ueber die medizinischen Folgezustände der Katastrophe von Courrières (10. März 06) unter eingehender Berücksichtigung der ursächlichen Momente mit vergleichenden Beobachtungen über die Katastrophe von Hamm (12. Nov. 08) und die Erdbeben von Valparaiso (16. Aug. 06) und Süditalien (28. Dez. 08)". This work made a significant contribution to psychiatry. Stierlin wrote about psycho-neurotic conditions of the survivors of the disasters. He visited the accident sites of Courrieres, Valparaiso and Messina and was able to understand as almost no one else, the souls of the survivors.

Preparing this work he researched the physical-chemical background of coal dust explosion. His knowledge about the causes and results of these catastrophes was so extensive and thorough that the common opinion was that he had studied mining as well as medicine. In his travels Stierlin displayed an excellent grasp of diplomacy which he employed successfully in Courrieres (where the mining organization tried to hide the true circumstances of the accident). This monograph on the aftermath of major catastrophes, written by a young doctor, became a classic and Stierlin is often mentioned until these days as a prominent Swiss psychiatrist.

After a long period of study in internal medicine in the hospitals of St. Gallen, Eppendorf and Zurich, he became an assistant at the surgical university clinic of de Quervain in Basel.

Being a skilled surgeon, in October 1912 Stierlin went to Serbia with 2 other Basel surgeons - Christoph A. Socin and Adolf L. Vischer. They were the only foreign Red Cross doctors to be allowed to go to the front lines of the 1st Balkan War at the time of the battle of Monastir. They worked in Serbian hospitals, exposed to sufferings and disasters of the war. In February 1913 as a chief of the Swiss Red Cross expedition Stierlin went again to the Balkan war. There he contracted a severe case of typhus fever which would later be the cause of a serious chronic heart disease and probably contributed to his early death.

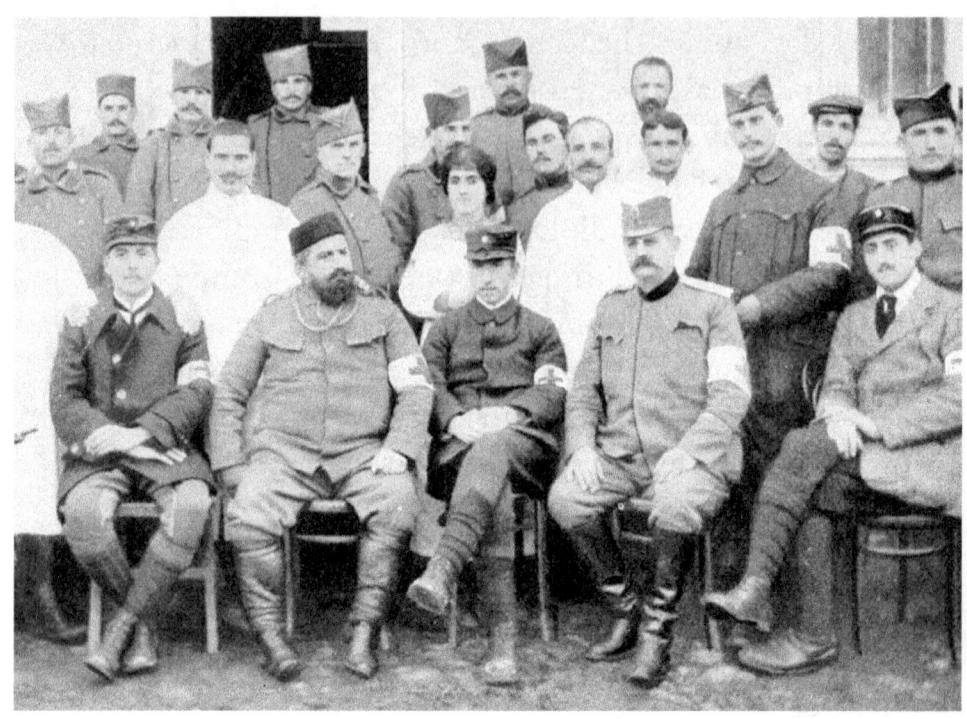

Eduard Stierlin (sitting in the center) with the staff of Monastir hospital.

From the fall of 1914 he worked as an assistant and later as a chief surgeon of Ernst Ferdinand Sauerbruch in the Kantonspital in Zurich. His work with Sauerbruch, who would become one of the greatest surgeons of the 20th century, proved to have the decisive effect on his surgical career. Despite their differences in temperament, Sauerbruch and Stierlin shared a common trait towards the extraordinary, and largesse united them.

Over the years Stierlin acquired such a high

profile position as a lecturer in Zurich, that everyone tried to persuade Stierlin to stay and not to follow Sauerbruch to Munich.

However, when in the fall of 1918 Sauerbruch asked Stierlin to accompany him to work at the University of Munich, Stierlin's short answer was: "if I can help you, of course!"

Stierlin's life was very compressed and included work, disappointments, hopes, sadness and a carefree love of life. Stierlin was a highly talented and well-educated surgeon. He was marked by an excellent ability of scientific observation. He loved surgery because he was able to help people, but more than that, because surgery brought him truth and clarity.

Stierlin was an unusual case of the skilled surgeon and prominent psychiatrist who developed the entire discipline of trauma and fear neuroses. Stierlin's investigations on stomach and intestinal activity are known, as are his works on the functional disturbances of the large intestine, on the mobile cecum, ulcerative colitis, osteitis fibrosa and the pharmacological studies on the influence of opiates on motility of the gastro-intestinal tract. He wrote a handbook on the clinical roentgen diagnosis of the intestinal tract which was unmatched in thoroughness and reliability in his time. He also completed the work about the roentgen diagnosis of the pathology of the thorax. He studied the pathology of the peptic ulcer from the (then) new

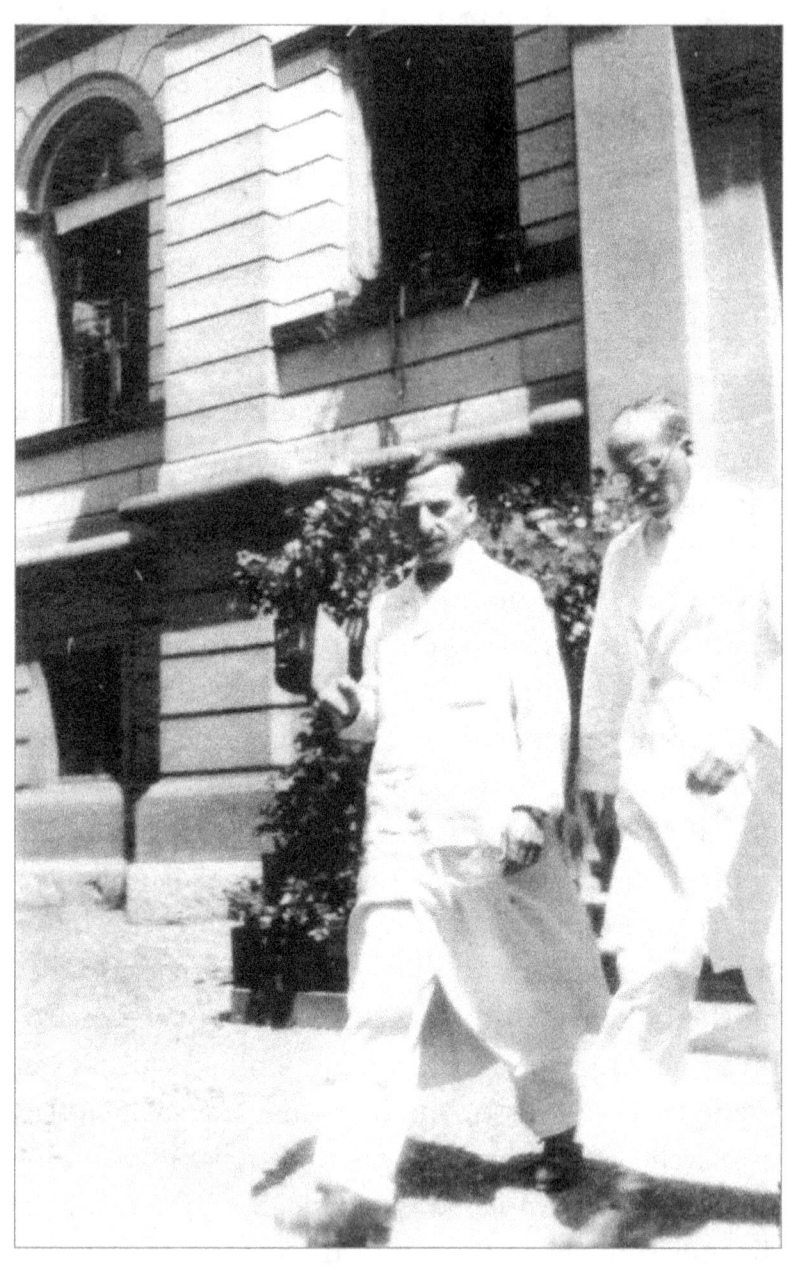

*Eduard Stierlin and Ferdinand Sauerbruch
when they worked at Kantonsspital in Zurich.*

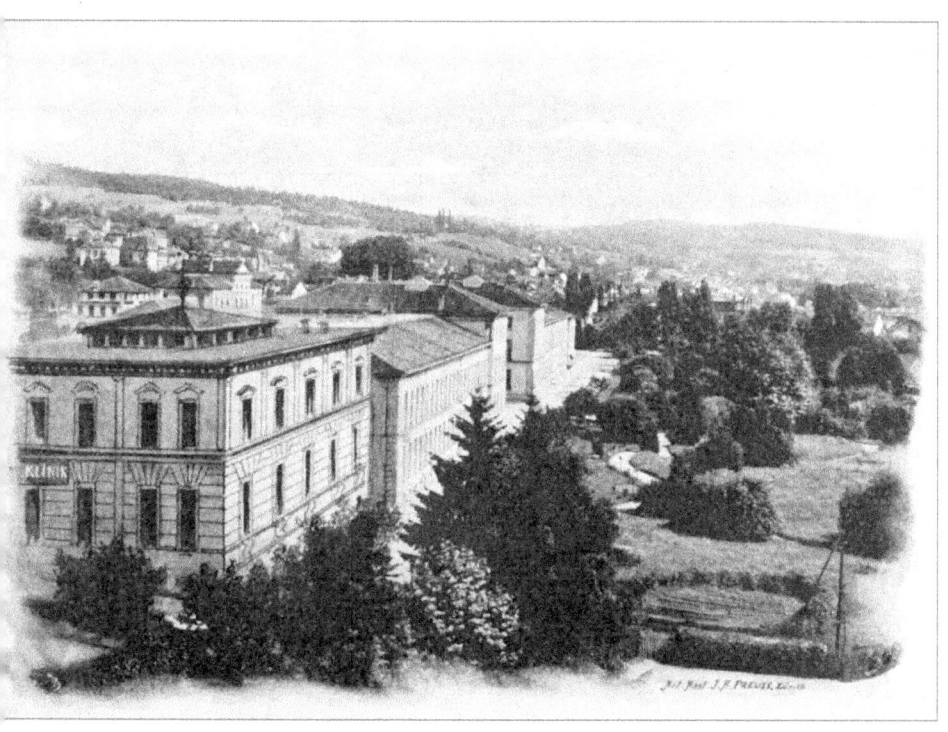

|| *Kantonsspital, Zurich.*

viewpoint, examining the significance of the vagus and sympathetic nerves.

In 1911 Stierlin described radiographic changes in tuberculosis involving ileum and cecum.

From the article published by P.F.Moller in 1922 and named "Roentgen Examination of Ileocaecal Tuberculosis with Special Reference to the so-called Stierlin-Sign" it appears that Stierlin sign had been commonly used in the medical literature of the 1910s.

In Munich, in the large clinical center, Stierlin's

Aus der chirurgischen Universitätsklinik Basel (früher Professor Wilms, jetzt Professor de Quervain).

Die Radiographie in der Diagnostik der Ileozoekaltuberkulose und anderer Krankheiten des Dickdarms*).

Von Dr. Eduard Stierlin, Assistent der Klinik.

Es ist eine bekannte Tatsache, dass die Ileozoekaltuberkulose, namentlich in ihren Anfangsstadien, der Diagnostik oft erhebliche Schwierigkeiten bereitet. Besonders häufig sind Verwechslungen mit den verschiedenen Formen der chronischen Appendizitis, Typhlitis, Kolitis. Aber auch die verschiedensten anderen abdominalen Erkrankungen sind schon gelegentlich durch eine Ileozoekaltuberkulose vorgetäuscht worden, besonders in den Stadien der Krankheit, wo man noch keinen Tumor fühlt. Die diagnostische Schwierigkeit wird durch die häufige Abwesenheit anderer manifester tuberkulöser Herde im Körper erhöht.

Ein neues diagnostisches Hilfsmittel zur Erkennung dieser frühen Stadien der Ileozoekaltuberkulose mag deshalb Chirurgen und Internisten gleich willkommen sein. Es wird uns von der Radiographie geboten. In einer Reihe von solchen klinisch unklaren Fällen ist es uns in letzter Zeit möglich gewesen, Strikturen im unteren Ileumende, sowie indurierende und ulzeröse Prozesse in der Wand des Zoekums und Colon ascendens mit dieser Methode festzustellen und so der Diagnose den richtigen Weg zu weisen.

das Colon ascendens in wechselnder [Aus...] tiefen Schatten und enthalten oft säu[...] Verengerung des Dünndarms in seine[n] muss also in einer 6 Stunden nach [...] gemachten Aufnahme am sichersten zu [...]

Ich lasse hier gleich das wesentlich[...] geschichte von einem der 2 erwähnten [...]

Es handelt sich um einen 25 jährigen M[...] nährungszustand. Vor ungefähr 4 Jahren [...] krankte er ziemlich akut an sehr heftigen [...] unteren Bauchgegend und lag 2 Wochen [...] zwischen 37 und 38°. Kein Erbrechen. Stuhl[...] später unterzog er sich der Appendektomie [...] zog sich infolge langen Bestehens einer eite[...] Erst ein Jahr nach der Operation schloss [...] In der Zeit erkrankte Patient an einer Lunge[...] dann 5 Monate wegen Lungenspitzenkatarr[...] Anfangs des Jahres 1908 (also vor ca. 2½ [...] plötzlich sehr heftige Kolikschmerzen in und [...] gegend, die 2—3 Stunden dauerten. Kein Erbre[...] Diese Schmerzattacken wiederholten sich alle [...] und wieder mit Brechreiz und Brechen ver[...] mählich länger. Nach Windabgang trat häuf[...] schmerzzeit fühlte sich Pat. vollkommen wohl, [...] alle Tage normalen Stuhlgang. Der letzte A[...] statt. Die Schmerzen dauerten damals 5 Tag[...] abhängig vom Essen, nachmittags oder abe[...] auf.

Pat. kommt unter der Wahrscheinl[...]

Original article by Eduard Stierlin in Münchner Medizinische Wochenschrift, 1911.

nature, which was always directed towards bigger things, found its true field of action. The difficult times of the revolution and disorder couldn't change this neutral Swiss, who remained always calm. People knew Stierlin as "sichere Punkt an den man sich halten konnte" – reliable to the very end. He was the soul of the Munich Surgical Clinic, where he was liked so much that its expression during his last illness surprised even himself.

Stierlin was a stimulating and thorough teacher, a

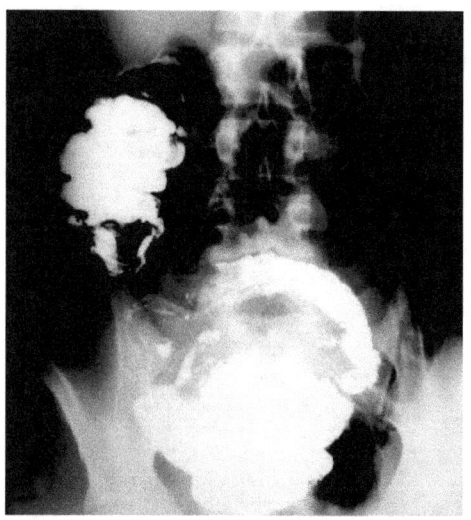

Stierlin sign –terminal ileum empties directly into stenotic ascending colon with non-opacification of the fibrotic and contracted cecum in tuberculous involvement of the ileocecum*

caring and sympathetic doctor. As chief surgeon, he was strict but just, a counselor and assistant to his younger colleagues. He alleviated the heavy burden of the nurses and had full understanding for their tasks.

For Stierlin, a Swiss, it was surely not easy to leave his fatherland and give up his good position in the Zurich clinic during the war years. He went to Germany at the climax of the unrest and despair of the fall of 1918. He did so being convinced that in the larger working arena he would have further opportunities for development.

The few free hours which he had, Stierlin devoted to the arts. He loved music and practiced it himself. He also found time to read good books. With friends he was the funniest man who delighted others with his sense of humor.

Eduard Stierlin †*).

Hochverehrte Anwesende!

Am 6. November früh ist mein langjähriger Oberarzt, Mitarbeiter und Freund, Prof. Dr. Eduard Stierlin, an den Folgen eines schweren Herzleidens gestorben. Kaum 1 Jahr durfte er der Münchener Hochschule angehören und hier Lehrer der Chirurgie sein. Er starb im 42. Lebensjahre.

Als Sohn eines Ingenieurs wurde Stierlin in der Schweiz geboren. Seinen Vater verlor er früh. Mit den Geschwistern und der treusorgenden Mutter verlebte er trotzdem eine sonnige Jugend in Zürich. Nach bestandenem Abiturientenexamen widmete er sich dem Maschinenbau, musste aber diesen Beruf aufgeben weil er ihm körperlich nicht gewachsen war.

Er studierte dann Medizin in Basel und Zürich und machte 1903 das Staatsexamen. Nach langer Ausbildung in der inneren Medizin an den Krankenhäusern in St. Gallen, Eppendorf und Zürich wurde er Assistent an der chirurgischen Universitätsklinik in Basel.

Im ersten Balkankrieg leitete er die schweizerische Expedition und zog sich im ärztlichen Dienste eines schweren Flecktyphus zu. Dieser gab den Anstoss zu einer schweren chronischen Herzerkrankung, die Stierlins frühen Tod bedingte. Im Januar 1915 kam er als erster Assistent an die Klinik nach Zürich und wurde bald Oberarzt. Hier blieb er, bis wir gemeinsam im vorigen Herbst nach München übersiedelten.

In diesem Rahmen drängt sich sein Leben zusammen. Arbeit, Enttäuschungen, Hoffnungen, Trauer und sonnige Lebensfreude.

Stierlin war ein hochbegabter und allgemein durchgebildeter Arzt, aber in dem sicheren einer, für seinen Spezialberuf — die Chirurgie — weitgehende Vorbedingungen mit sich brachte. Ihn zeichnete eine hervorragende naturwissenschaftliche Beobachtungsgabe aus, die, wie v. Bergmann einmal sagte, gerade für den Chirurgen mehr wert ist als Talent und Kunst. Er liebte die Chirurgie, weil er den Leuten helfen konnte, vor allen Dingen aber, weil sie ihm Wahrheit und Klarheit schaffte.

Schon als junger Mediziner schuf er grundlegende Arbeiten. Unter ihnen ist in erster Linie seine klassische Monographie über die Folgen grosser Katastrophen zu nennen. Mit zäher Ausdauer hat er die Unfallstätten in Courrières, Valparaiso und in Messina bereist und in den Seelen der das Unglück Ueberlebenden zu lesen verstanden, wie kaum ein anderer. Die Ergebnisse seiner Arbeit sind befruchtend für die ganze Lehre der traumatischen und Schreckneurosen gewesen.

In reiferen Jahren haben ihn eine Reihe von Fragen aus der allgemeinen Pathologie und der chirurgischen Klinik beschäftigt. Bekannt sind seine Untersuchungen der Magen-Darmtätigkeit. Seine Arbeiten über die Funktionsstörungen des Dickdarms, über das Coecum mobile, die Colitis ulcerosa, über die Ostitis fibrosa und die pharmakologischen Untersuchungen über den Einfluss von Morphium, Opium und Pantopon auf die Bewegungen des Magendarmkanals.

Sein Handbuch über die klinische Röntgendiagnostik des Verdauungskanals ist an Gründlichkeit und Zuverlässigkeit der Beobachtungen bisher unerreicht. Eine weitere, gemeinsam mit Chaoul gerade beendete, zusammenfassende Darstellung der Pathologie der ThoraxThoraxorgane im Röntgenbild wird in der Folge befruchtend wirken. Ueber den engen Rahmen der Röntgendiagnostik hinaus werden darin pathologisch-anatomische Befunde und klinische Fragestellungen eingehend gewürdigt. In der allerletzten Zeit hat der rastlose Mann die Pathologie des Ulcus ventriculi von neuen Gesichtspunkten aus studiert und die Bedeutung des Vagus und Sympathikus für die physiologische und pathologische Sekretion der Nieren in durchaus origineller Weise untersucht. Es war ihm ein tröstender Gedanke, dass diese letzte, ihm ans Herz gewachsene Arbeit eben beendet werden konnte. Alle Untersuchungen zeichnen sich durch Zuverlässi... Als f... Wissen e... zustellen... richtiger...

und Berater in persönlichen Dingen. So kam es, dass die Klinik auch in der schwersten Zeit auf ihn bauen konnte. Als ich nach meiner Berufung hierher ihn fragte, ob er mit mir gehen wollte, war seine kurze Antwort; Wenn ich Ihnen helfen kann, selbstverständlich. Es war für ihn als Schweizer sicher nicht leicht, sein Vaterland und seine schöne Stelle an der Zürcher Klinik in Kriegszeiten aufzugeben. Er tat es dennoch in der Ueberzeugung, dass er in dem grösseren Arbeitsfeld weitere Entwicklungsmöglichkeiten habe und dass er es sich selbst schuldig war. Auch Anhänglichkeit und Freude an unserer gemeinsamen Arbeit hat ihn wohl mitbestimmt.

In dieser Trauerstunde will ich ihm noch einmal danken für die Treue, die er mir gehalten hat und mit der er in einer schweren politischen Krise in der Schweiz, die in meiner Abwesenheit im Fekte über die Klinik hereinbrach, mit offenem Visier, ohne seine eigene Person und Ehre zu schonen, für seinen Chef und seine Klinik eintrat.

Auch seit ihm unvergessen, wie er als Schweizer die Not unseres Vaterlandes miltempfunden und für unser Land gelitten hat. Er hatte begriffen, wie sein grosser Landsmann Gottfried Keller, dass trotz aller politischen und nationalen Grenzen die deutsche Schweiz dieselbe Sprache spricht wie Deutschland und dass über alle Hindernisse hinweg die Stimme des Blutes mächtiger sein sollte als politische und wirtschaftliche Interessen. Und trotz allem Schwsssslichen und Niederdrückenden, was er in der Revolution in unserem Vaterlande sah, hat er den Glauben an Deutschlands Wiederentwicklung nicht verloren und sich gefreut, dass er die ersten Spuren davon noch miterleben konnte.

Die wenigen Freistunden, die ihm seine rastlose praktische und wissenschaftliche Tätigkeit übrig liess, widmete er der Kunst. Stierlin liebte die Musik und übte sie selbst aus. Er fand daneben noch Zeit, gute Bücher zu lesen, mit besonderer Liebe seine Landsleute Gottfried Keller und Konrad Ferdinand Meyer.

Im Kreise seiner Freunde wich die sonst ihm eigentümliche Reserve. Er war der Vergnügtesten einer und hat uns mit seinem goldenen Humor oft erfreut.

Es würde das Bild Stierlins unvollständig sein, wollte man nicht seines herzlichen Verhältnisses zu seiner Mutter und seinen Geschwistern gedenken. Mit rührender Liebe hat er an ihnen gehangen und im regen Verkehr mit ihnen Land er Kraft zu neuer Arbeit.

In dieser schweren Zeit, in der persönliche Schicksale zurücktreten müssen gegenüber grossen Geschehnissen, die uns umgeben, verliert vielleicht der Tod eines Einzelnen an Bedeutung. Wir aber, die von ihm so hart betroffen werden, fühlen die Lücke, die er hinterlässt, schwer.

Stierlin selbst sah seinen Tod kommen. Er hat sich gegen ihn gewehrt, weil er das Leben liebte. Als er aber fühlte, dass jener stärker sei, hat er ihm tapfer ins Auge geschaut. Noch vor allen hat er warmen Abschied genommen.

Die Anerkennung der Fakultät, die ihm in der Ernennung als Professor zum Ausdruck gebracht wurde, die vielen Beweise der Liebe und Anhänglichkeit, die er in diesem Hause während seiner schweren Krankheit erhielt, waren seine letzten grossen Freuden und haben ihm den Schluss seines Lebens wundervoll umrahmt.

Mitten aus der Arbeit und aus erfolgreichem Schaffen riss ihn ein hartes Geschick. Aber es versöhnte ihn das beglückende Gefühl, durch den frühen Tod ein wertvolles Leben beendet zu haben.

Mir haben die Worte Konrad Ferdinand Meyers ein, die er den sterbenden Ulrich v. Hutten sagen lässt:

Ich reise, Freund. Ein Boot, ich reise weit.
Mein letztes Wort, ein Wort der Dankbarkeit.

F. Sauerbruch.

Et puisque le calcul des probabilités nous donne le moyen de le faire, nous pouvons dire qu'il représente tout au moins une méthode qui se laisse fort bien soutenir et qui est même basée sur des arguments singulièrement concluants. Je crois que chacun doit se déclarer d'accord avec cette formule conciliante. C'est intentionnellement que je me suis retenu de dire que cette méthode était indispensable.

Varia.

Prof. Dr. med. Eduard Stierlin †.

Am 6. November 1919 starb in München Dr. med. Eduard Stierlin. Nur für kurze Zeit war es ihm vergönnt, in seiner neuen, aussichtsreichen Stellung als Oberarzt an der Münchner chirurgischen Universitätsklinik die mit grosser Freude und Begeisterung übernommene Arbeit zu vollbringen.

Eduard Stierlin wurde 1878 in Zürich geboren, besuchte die Zürcher Schulen und wandte sich ursprünglich den Maschinentechnik zu; später erst studierte er in Zürich, Bern, Berlin, Hamburg und Tübingen Medizin und promovierte in Zürich mit einer vielbeachteten Arbeit „Ueber psychoneuropathische Folgeerscheinungen der Gefangenschaft der Katastrophe von Cour... Nach... mit Prof. Sauerbruch an die chirurgische Universitätsklinik nach München.

Stierlin war weit in der Welt herumgekommen. Gleich nach seinem Staatsexamen reiste er als Schiffsarzt nach Südamerika. Seine Studien führten ihn später nach Belgien, Frankreich und Italien. Anregend und oftmals mit köstlichem Humor wußte er zu erzählen von seinem abwechslungsreichen Reiseleben oder auch von seinen interessanten Erlebnissen auf dem Balkankriegsschauplatz, wo er im Winter 1912/13 als Kriegschirurg tätig war. Damals erkrankte Stierlin im Lazarett von Durasso an Flecktyphus, von dessen Folgen, einem Pleuraempyem, er sich erst nach langdauerndem, mit Humor und viel Geduld ertragenem Krankenlager erholte. Schon damals gab der Zustand seines Herzens wiederholt zu Besorgnis Veranlassung. Eine schwere Grippe, die Stierlin im vergangenen Herbst durchmachte, mag vielleicht auch dazu beigetragen haben, seine Widerstandskraft so zu schwächen, daß er nun, im Alter von 41 Jahren, einem Herzleiden erliegen mußte. Lüdin.

Vereinsberichte.

Sitzung der Schweiz. Aerzte-Kommission.

Samstag und Sonntag, den 22./23. November 1919. Im Hotel Schweizerhof, in Bern.

Obituaries at E.Stierlin's death from Münchner Medizinische Wochenschrift (written by Ferdinand Sauerbruch) and from Schweizerische Medizinische Wochenschrift.

On November 6, 1919 in Munich, Germany, Stierlin died at the age of 42 as a result of serious heart disease precipitated at the disastrous second wave of Spanish flu. Just in the evening before finally succumbing to his illness he finished three new works. During his illness he received the news that he had been promoted to extraordinary Professor. He had worked as a chief surgeon and professor at University of Munich for not even a year. ◆

Thomas Terry Hoar-Stevens

"Filling the Gap"

Terry-Thomas sign is a widening of the scapho-lunate interval. This sign was not named after the person who described it. Victor H. Frankel, orthopedic surgeon from Seattle, suggested in 1977 to apply the anthropomorphic sign of dental diastema (gap between the upper incisors) to aid in the recognition of rotatory subluxation of the scaphoid bone of the wrist. It is also the chronologically latest eponym introduced into radiology practice. Terry-Thomas himself permitted the use of his name as a mnemonic aid for rotational subluxation of the scaphoid. It was a wise decision, since the use of the radiological sign may even outlive the actor's fame, who is frequently unknown to younger generations. Even the name of

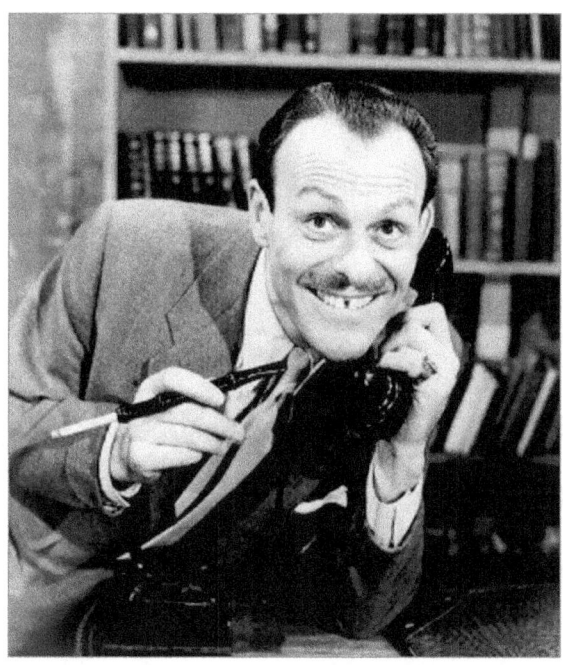

Gap between the upper incisors (dental diastema) of Terry-Thomas.

Terry-Thomas' autobiography "Filling the Gap" could provide orthopedic surgeons with a clue as to the treatment: the gap is filled by rotating the scaphoid and fixing it with pins or a cast.

Terry-Thomas was born as Thomas Terry Hoar-Stevens in Finchley, England on July 14, 1911. He worked as a clerk before going into show business. Drifting from cabaret to background actor in the movies he found success as an entertainer during World War II. After the war, he worked in TV and radio becoming in the mid-1950s famous in TV

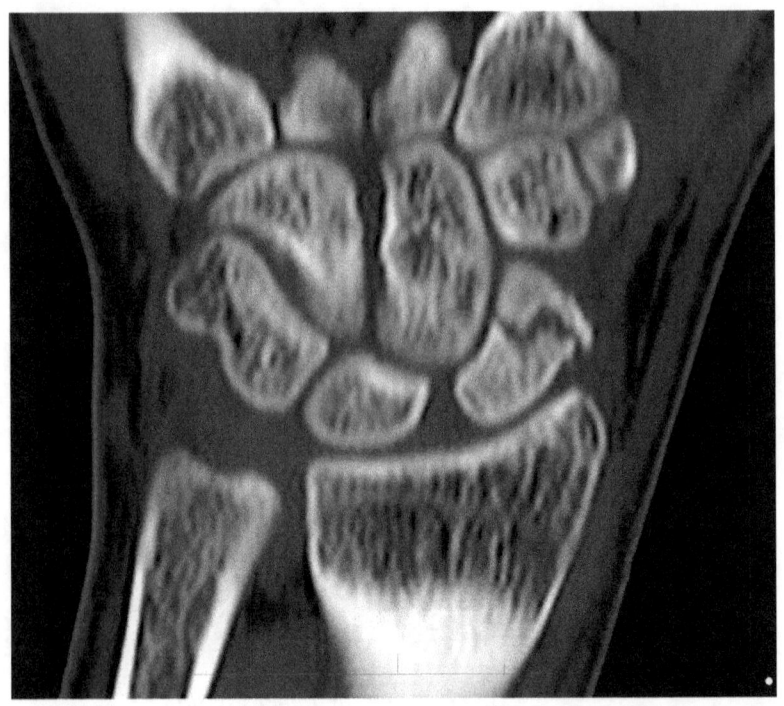

Terry-Thomas sign of widening of scapholunate interval.
Note the associated scaphoid fracture.

series and in movies. He also had a gifted voice with a range of accents in his repertoire. He wanted to change his name from Thomas Stevens to the stage name Thomas Terry, but feared that this might be taken as an attempt to pass himself off as a relation of the actress Ellen Terry. Thus he reversed it to Terry Thomas. In 1948, he added a hyphen between the two names in order to be more distinctive, to stop people calling him "Mr. Thomas" which he disliked.

Terry-Thomas became famous for his portrayal of the archetypal cad, bounder and absolute rotter. In 1966, he played a notable but very different role as an RAF airman in the French film La Grande Vadrouille, which for over 40 years remained the most successful film in the history of cinema in France. Diagnosed in 1971 with Parkinson's disease, Terry-Thomas retired by 1977.

He died on January 8, 1990 in Busbridge Hall nursing home in Godalming, England. ◆

Nils Johan Hugo Westermark

Silver Medal in Sailing in the Olympic Games

Westermark sign is an appearance of pulmonary ischemia in pulmonary embolism as a clarified area with diminished vascular design corresponding to the extent of the embolised artery. The vascularisation which is maintained in the central parts of the lung takes, however, a rapid end to pass over into the above mentioned area of non-vascularisation.

Nils Johan Hugo Westermark was born in Stockholm, Sweden on September 9, 1892. He finished college in Stockholm in 1911 and got his MD in 1919 graduating from Karolinska Institute Medical School. In 1920-1921 he worked as a radiologist in Sabbatsbergs hospital and in 1922-1923 in Karolinska Radium Hospital (Radiumhemmet). From 1923 until

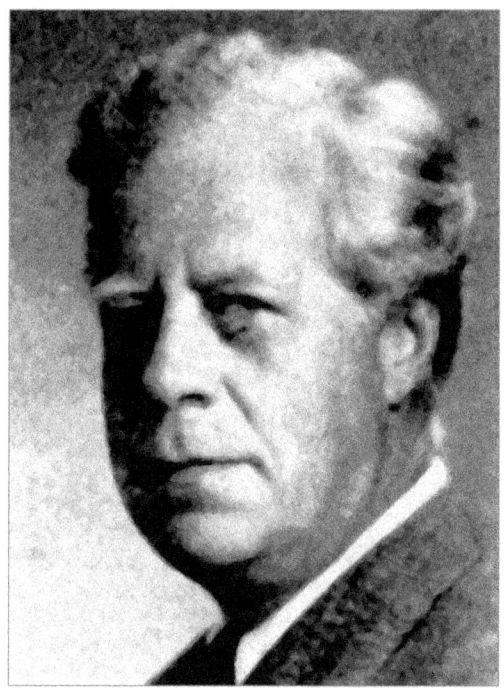

Nils Johan Hugo Westermark *

1929 he worked at St. Eriks hospital. Westermark received his PhD in Medicine (Radiology) in 1930. In 1930 he came to St. Görans Hospital, Stockholm and stayed there until 1957.

He was appointed Dozent at Karolinska Institute in 1930 and Professor in 1955.

He was a member of the board in the Swedish Society of Medical Radiology 1928-57, and a member of the Nordic Society of Medical Radiology from 1928-53. He was internationally active, and was an official Swedish delegate at several international

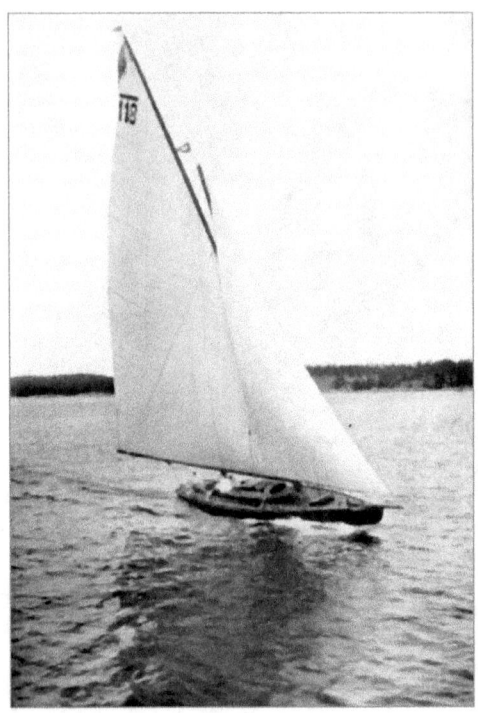

Sans Atout at 1912 Summer Olympics.

radiology conferences. He presented the first Rigler lecture at University of Minnesota in 1946 and held a Mayo Foundation lecture in 1946.

In 1912 Nils Westermark was part of the Swedish team which took the silver medal in sailing the boat *Sans Atout* at the competition of 8 metre class in the Vth Olympic Games in Stockholm. His brother, Herbert Westermark, a gynecologist and Marine physician, was on the same winning team. Interestingly, in the article in Wikipedia, Nils Westermark is described only as a Swedish sailor who competed in the 1912

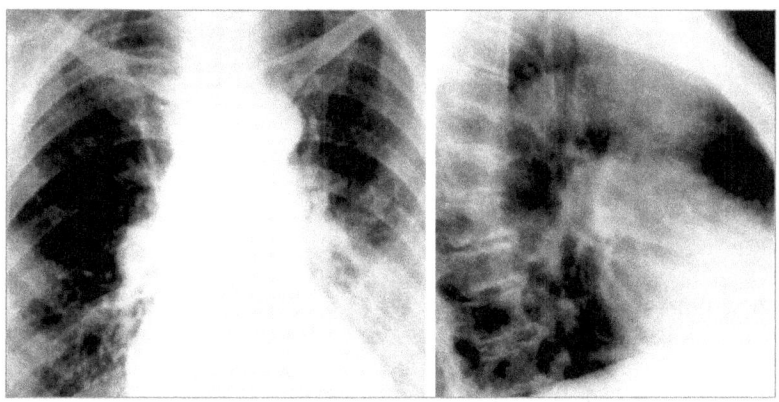

Westermark sign of oligemia and abrupt ending of the pulmonary vessels*

Summer Olympics without mention of his career as a radiologist.

In 1938, Westermark described the appearance of pulmonary embolism on x-ray, writing: "In embolism of the pulmonary artery without infarction we get ischaemia of the branches of the pulmonary artery on the peripheral side of the embolus. On the radiogram this ischaemia appears as a clarified area with diminished vascular design corresponding to the extent of the embolised artery. The vascularisation is however maintained in the central parts of the lung. The vascularisation takes however a rapid end to pass over into the above mentioned area of non-vascularisation".

Nils Johan Hugo Westermark died on January 24, 1980 in Stockholm. ◆

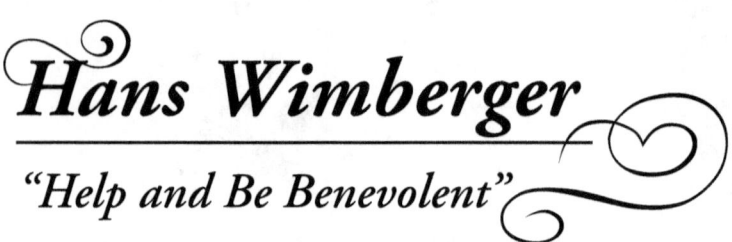

Hans Wimberger

"Help and Be Benevolent"

The Hunt for Hans Wimberger

Two radiological eponyms carry the name of Wimberger. Wimberger sign refers to bilateral metaphyseal destruction in the medial proximal tibias seen in congenital syphilis. Wimberger ring is a sclerotic ring around the epiphysis indicating loss of epiphyseal density in children with scurvy.

Ambiguity surrounded the identity of the person who described these signs. Medcyclopaedia indicates that it was the German radiologist, Heinrich Wimberger. However, a literature search revealed the article signed H. Wimberger and several articles signed Hans Wimberger published in the 1920s and dedicated to the diagnosis

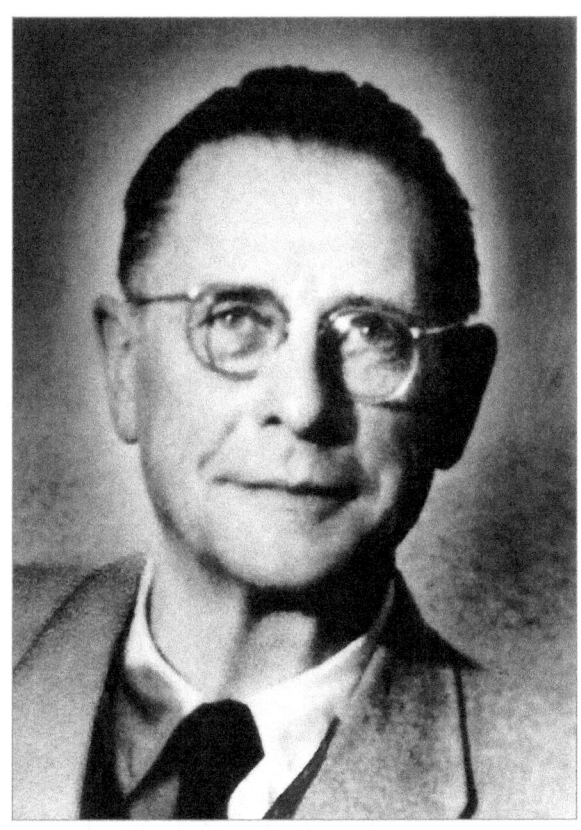

Hans Wimberger. Previously unpublished photograph from the family archives. Courtesy of Gerhard Wimberger.

of rickets, syphilis and scurvy in children. We found that Hans Wimberger was a physician who worked in Universitäts-Kinderklinik located at Lazarettgasse 14 in Vienna, Austria. We were able to find references to Hans Wimberger in Austrian newspapers and in the report of the Lister Institute in London, England. In "The work of the accessory food factors committee", Hans Wimberger was mentioned as a distinguished x-ray specialist at the Kinderklinik. Hans Wimberger had an appointment as Dozent in Universitäts-Kinderklinik and published several articles on the diagnosis of rickets, scurvy, and syphilis in children.

From the Landesarchiv of Salzburg we learned that Hans Christoph Wimberger was born on June 26, 1887 in Bischofshofen (Land Salzburg), Austria. He was a son of a railway engineer. He died on October 16, 1954 in Salzburg, Austria.

From the newspaper "Klinische Wochenschrift" of July 23, 1927, we found that Dr. Hans Wimberger, Assistant Professor at the Universitäts-Kinderklinik in Vienna, became the Primararzt (chief physician) of the Children's Department at the Landeshospital in Salzburg.

Attempts to find relatives of Hans Wimberger among people with the same last name in his native town of Bischofshofen failed. None of those whom we contacted knew about a Dr. Hans Wimberger among their ancestors or relatives.

We were advised that Dr. Gerhart Harrer would be able to provide us with details about Hans Wimberger. This was really mysterious. What did the infamous Nazi psychiatrist have in common with the radiologist? Anyway, we did not receive a reply from this direction.

However, we noticed that one of the Wimbergers in Salzburg, Gerhard Wimberger, professor of music, famous composer and conductor, was born in Vienna in 1923 and had moved to Salzburg by 1940. Understanding that kids usually do not travel alone and matching it with the period when Hans Wimberger took his position in Salzburg, we realized that these facts might be very relevant. We called Gerhard Wimberger and after telling him that we were looking for Hans Wimberger, we heard "Ja, das war mein Vater" – yes, this was my father.

Professor Gerhard Wimberger and later his brother, Dr. Herbert Wimberger, (a psychiatrist in Washington, USA) provided us with details about their father. We are happy to be the first to publish biographical details about Dr. Hans Wimberger who is to be credited for the description of the sign and the ring named after him.

Hans Wimberger was born on June 26, 1887 in Bischofshofen (Land Salzburg), Austria in the small building near the tracks. His father was a "Heizhausoberkommisar" who was in charge of the condition and readiness of the steam engines at the nodal point in Bischofshofen where four railway lines intersected: the main East-West line through Austria, one heading east through the "Ennstal" and one climbing to the tunnel crossing the Alps into southern Austria. When Hans was 16 years old his father, who had been a heavy smoker, died, probably of a heart attack.

Initially, Hans was not a good student at the grade

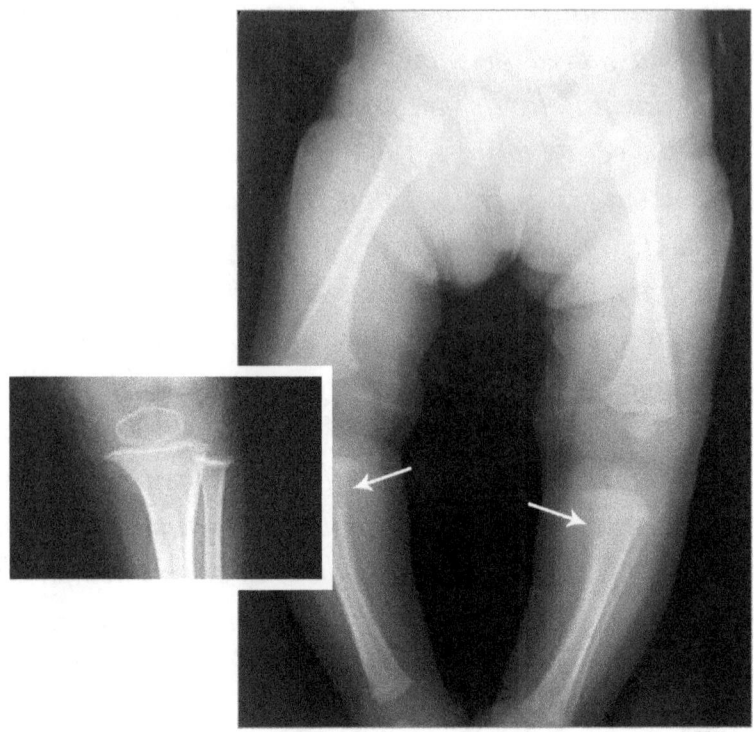

Wimberger sign - localized bony destruction of the medial portion of the proximal tibial metaphysis in congenital syphilis*
Wimberger ring – sclerotic ring around epiphysis indicating loss of epiphyseal density in scurvy*

school in Bischofshofen and failed second grade. His strict, no-nonsense rather humorless mother, Babette, did not let him come home for Christmas. 11 year old Hans went to the railroad station and sat there on a bench and cried. After repeating second grade, he did well at school and entered the Gymnasium in Salzburg.

Young Hans spent a lot of time hiking and traveling. As the son of a railroad employee he had a free pass on the railroad. He was also a spelunker exploring the limestone mountains which had extensive cave systems. On one of these trips, he discovered a subterranean waterfall, which still carries his name – "Johannisfall" (Johann is the full form of Hans) in the Tennengebirge.

During the winter months, Hans was one of the early skiers. Skiing was then still in its infancy. Hans carried the crudely shaped wooden boards, with leather straps for holding the leather hiking boots in place, up to the high farms dotting the steep hillsides, or, using skins strapped to the underside of the boards, climbing up to a mountain top. There were no prepared runs, and certainly no lifts. The skier descended in deep snow, carving elegant turns using the "telemark" technique. For the rest of his life Hans Wimberger preferred the deep snow over the skied-out runs when he skied.

After, and even before his father's death, two men figured strongly in his life. One was "uncle August" - Dr. August Heinrich, his father's best friend, an avid naturalist and traveler. Hans's father and August Heinrich met and married the sisters Maurer – Babette and Katharina in 1870. Another was retired Professor Hans Crammer who lived in a beautiful mountain valley in the village of Mühlbach west of Bischofshofen. Visiting him, Hans went on a hike with a few of Crammer's relatives. Coming back from the hike he happened to carry on his shoulders a little 7 year old girl, Gretl (short for Margarete) who had become tired. This would have an important implication on his later life.

During those years Hans became interested in photography, organizing his own darkroom for developing the photographs.

After passing the "Matura", the final examination after the eight years of Gymnasium, Hans went to the Medical School of the University of Graz. He joined "Akademischer Turnverein", the student fraternity with the focus on gymnastics and physical exercise.

He received his MD shortly before the outbreak of WWI. Hans Wimberger served in the Austro-Hungarian army as military physician initially on the Italian front in the Dolomites. He distinguished himself as a leader and was transferred to Sofia, Bulgaria where he was in charge of the military hospital. There he was noticed by Professor Anton Eiselsberg, the military physician in charge of the southern front who had been a famous professor of surgery in Vienna. Eiselsberg's recommendation after the war helped an unemployed doctor to find work. Eiselsberg's cousin, Clemens von Pirquet, Professor of Pediatrics at the University of Vienna, accepted Hans Wimberger in 1919 as an assistant at his Kinderklinik.

(Aus der Universitäts-Kinderklinik in Wien [Vorstand: Prof. Dr. *Cl. Pirquet*].)

Über die Ätiologie der Rachitis im Säuglingsalter[1]).

Beobachtungen über ~~. (Bei~~ und Heilung.

Harriette Chick, ~~Son Smith, R. R.~~ Hume, Helen
M. M. Mackay ~~~~ H. Hender-

Unter Mitarbeit von

Dr. Hans Wimberger,

Vorläuf ~~~~ Röntgenologen ~~ster-

der Universitäts-Kinderklinik.

Die ~~*Accessory Food Factors Commit*~~ ellen
einen Au s *Medical Research Council.* hrten
Untersuch ht auf
die ganze ~~~~ ht not-
wendigerweis ~~dungen im Text.~~ ehmen
wird, hielten w n-
zeit zu veröffentl ~~14. Juli 1922~~ n
erhaltenen Resultate, Schluss e
lassen möge.

Die Untersuchung war in der Hoffnung unternommen worden, definitive Lösung des Problems zu gewinnen, ob die Säuglingsrachitis auf eine fehlerhafte Diät oder auf andere ungünstige Umstände in der Umgebung zu beziehen sei und ob im ersteren Falle eine Beziehung zwischen dem Auftreten der Erkrankung und dem Mangel eines spezifischen Nahrungsbestandteiles, nämlich des A-Vitamins festgelegt werden könne.

In Wien boten sich nun besondere Vorteile für eine Arbeit dieser Art. Seit 1918 war die Rachitis in der Stadt weit verbreitet, und zwar höhergradige Fälle, dergestalt, daß sich reichlich Gelegenheit für das Studium dieser Krankheit ergab. Es ist klar, daß brauchbare klinische Untersuchungen, welche sich mit der Beziehung von Diät und Auftreten

---

[1]) Ist in englischer Sprache im *Lancet* vom 1. Juli 1922 erschienen.

|| *Article from 1922 by the group of authors, including Hans Wimberger, mistakenly credited as roentgenologist.*

(Aus der Universitäts-Kinderklinik in Wien. — Vorstand: Prof. Dr. *Cl. Pirquet.*)

Der Säuglingsskorbut in Wien 1916—1923.

Von

Hans Wimberger,
Assistenten der Klinik.

Mit 5 Abbildungen im Text.

(Eingegangen am 25. März 1924.)

Die Frage nach den auslösenden Ursachen des Morbus Möller-Barlow beansprucht in jedem Einzelfalle, noch mehr aber bei Massenerkrankungen innerhalb eines gewissen Zeitraumes in einem geschlossenen Ernährungsgebiet großes Interesse. So genau die Ätiologie des Skorbuts in klinischer und experimenteller Hinsicht umschrieben ist, so schwierig können die Bedingungen zu erklären sein, unter denen die Avitaminose manifest wird. Sicherlich muß der Boden zur Erkrankung durch die Mangelnahrung erst bereitet sein, der Zeitpunkt des Krankwerdens hängt von verschiedenen Zufälligkeiten ab. Diese können endogener Natur als „Disposition" oder exogener Natur sein, d. h. auf zufällige Erkrankungen, soziale Verhältnisse, vielleicht sogar auch meteorologische Ursachen zurückgeführt werden. Der Begriff der „Dysergie" (*Abels*) für den an C-Faktor verarmten Organismus hat viel für sich und will die eigenartige Verfassung des Organismus bezeichnen, bei der ein zufälliger Infekt den Skorbut plötzlich unter den verschiedensten Symptomen zum Krankheitsbilde erhebt.

Als die beiden Hauptträger der Skorbutätiologie möchte ich den spezifischen Nahrungsdefekt einerseits, die individuelle Disposition andererseits bezeichnen, die beide in ihrer gegenseitigen Stellung und Wirkung von verschiedenen Hilfsfaktoren bestimmt werden. Dabei überwiegt das eine Mal dieser, das andere Mal jener ätiologisch so bedeutend, daß einer von beiden fast ganz verdeckt wird. So kann der Skorbut bei keineswegs auffallendem C-Faktormangel im „geeigneten" Individuum ebenso schwer verlaufen, wie er bei schwerem Nahrungsdefekt am „ungeeigneten" Organismus überhaupt oder doch lange ausbleiben kann.

Diese und verwandte ätiologische Fragen haben den Anlaß dazu gegeben, eine nun wohl als abgeschlossen anzusehende Periode besonderer Häufung von Barlow-Fällen in den Jahren 1916—1923 im Stadt-

|| Original article by Hans Wimberger in 1924

In addition to their regular duties, all assistants had to develop some special interest. The early interest in photography made Wimberger almost a natural to act as a radiologist and he became competent in handling the radiology films. However, he was never trained to be a radiologist. Radiology was then in its infancy; the equipment was simple. Much work was done with fluoroscopy, and x-rays were either in negative form - as they are now - or copied into positives. The lead-gloves were not reliable, and Hans Wimberger developed a life-long disfiguration of a finger nail, attributed to a faulty glove and x-ray damage.

Following the defeat in WWI, life in post-WWI Vienna was difficult. Starvation caused multiple cases of malnutrition, including scurvy. This made the Lister Institute of Preventive Medicine in London send a group of scientists to Vienna. Participating in their study on avitaminosis, Hans Wimberger published articles where he described bony changes in scurvy, rickets and syphilis. Due to his x-ray experience Wimberger was so helpful to the scientists from the Lister Institute, that 34 years later Harriette Chick and Margaret Hume, members of that group wrote that the work of the Accessory Food Factors Committee was assisted by Hans Wimberger, a distinguished x-ray specialist at the Kinderklinik who was "an invaluable part of the hospitality offered, and one indispensable for satisfactory investigation" of the committee. His knowledge of radiology caused people to consider him a specialist and mistakenly call him "Röntgenologe Hans Wimberger".

Wimberger systematically studied the skeletal x-rays of the children. Specifically, he described the x-ray pictures of children with scurvy, rickets and congenital syphilis during the height of their illness, and the subsequent course during treatment. These publications gained him recognition in the German-speaking pediatric community. However, he was totally unaware of the international recognition until 1947. Then he learned in a letter from his old friend and colleague from the Kinderklinik, Karl Kassowitz, who had immigrated to the USA in 1923, that the "Wimberger Sign" and the "Wimberger Ring" had become eponyms in the USA and beyond, being first introduced by John Caffey in his textbook, "Pediatric X-ray Diagnosis", published in 1945.

Work in the Kinderklinik of Clemens von Pirquet was intensive, interesting and demanding. Von Pirquet was an outstanding researcher, the founder of modern immunology. He was also an excellent organizer and leader of the Kinderklinik. The spirit and the individuality of the world-renowned clinic resulted from its harmonious union of research institute, model hospital, educational facility, and intellectual center for social welfare where the care for the well-being of the child was the first concern. The nursing staff had an established reputation which was admired in other countries including England and the USA. Von Pirquet was active in furthering the development of a well-trained, intelligent staff of nurses with outstanding ethical and scientific qualifications.

Von Pirquet held Wimberger in high esteem and wanted him to seek a chairmanship at a German university. Shortly before his tragic death in 1929 (he and his wife committed double suicide) von Pirquet wrote a will in which he also expressed his wish for a succession at the Kinderklinik. He wrote: "the following of my pupils are able to succeed me", listing six names with Hans Wimberger being one of them.

Von Pirquet considered mountains just "Steinerhaufen" (heaps of stones), useless since no food could be grown there. But Wimberger loved the outdoors and spent Sundays bicycling and hiking in the vicinity of Vienna. He again met Gretl Seiser, whom he had carried on his shoulders when she was 7 years old. He loved her spirit and the two enjoyed playing 4-hand piano together. Soon they decided to get married. However, at that time, assistants at the clinic were supposed to be completely devoted to their work and be celibate. Luckily, von Pirquet was more liberal in his thinking than most "Professors" and granted Wimberger permission to marry. After their son was born, the young mother was even allowed to push the baby stroller on the park-like grounds of the Kinderklinik.

In 1927 Wimberger learned that the post of "Primarius" (head) of the Kinderspital in Salzburg was available. He struggled hard, trying to decide whether to stay in the academic world, as his chief, von Pirquet, wanted him to, or whether to lead in the management of a hospital, as he had done during WWI in Bulgaria. He confided later that he had not felt qualified to become a department chair, an "Ordinarius". He also wanted to return to his beloved Salzburg, the city and the province, to the mountains he had got to know from all his hikes in earlier years. There is no doubt that he certainly could have been an excellent chairman of a pediatric department in a university. However, would he have been happy, far away from his beloved mountains? No one will ever know.

Wimberger took on the task of directing the Kinderspital in Salzburg with his usual energy. The hospital had several large rooms, each for a number of children. The nursing care was provided by nuns, but there was no training facility for pediatric nurses.

Wimberger founded a school for pediatric nurses. He managed to raise the needed funds aided by a grateful parent of a patient who was on the city council

- "Stadtrat" - and through the Rockefeller Foundation. Aside from modernizing the old building, he added a 3-story wing with glassed-in cubicles.

Wimberger was heavily involved in public health issues, specifically in the prevention of rickets, a very common disease then, especially in the rural population, by organizing public distribution of Vitamin D, and in the prevention of iodine-deficiencies - cretinism - which was common before the introduction of iodized table salt.

While mornings and evenings were devoted to the hospital, the rest of the time was given to the private practice. His private clinic was part of their apartment on the fourth floor of a typical Austrian apartment building: the front faced a fairly quiet street, the back a garden, behind which ran the railroad line from Salzburg to Munich, a major thoroughfare. All tenants, the family and the patients became immune to the noise of the trains rattling by. The waiting room had some wooden benches and on the door leading to the "Ordination" - the examining room - one could read Wimberger's motto: "Hilfe, und sei gütig" ("Help, and be benevolent").

The practice of medicine in those days meant making home visits. Since Wimberger did not own a car until 1936, he traveled all over town on a 2-speed bike. In winter he would wind a thick rope around his tires for better traction. Once he was called to see a 7-months old girl with whooping cough. Thanks to his treatment the baby recovered. Some twenty years later she married his son Herbert.

World War II brought bombing of Salzburg by the allied forces. The hospital was partly evacuated, with two of the units being placed in schools and monasteries about 15 miles outside the city. Wimberger was on the road a lot, driving a small motorcycle to make his rounds.

Hans and Gretl Wimberger had three sons. The elder, Gerhard, after serving in the army in 1941-1945 became a famous professor of music in Salzburg. Another son, non-commissioned officer Hans Peter was killed on April 1, 1945. News of his death hit Dr. Hans Wimberger very hard. The third son – Dr. Herbert Wimberger - moved to the United States with the help of Hans's friend, Karl Kassowitz, and practiced psychiatry in Winthrop, state of Washington. In contrast to the other members of his family, he discovered his love for music only at the age of 63 years.

After the war, as one who had not been against the Nazi regime, Hans Wimberger had to resign his position in September 1945. He continued to work in his private clinic. In 1950 Hans Wimberger was elected president of the Salzburg Medical Association. He based his campaign on the word "Anständigkeit" (decency). He not only ran the organization but also created a program to provide for a pension plan for retired physicians.

Hans Wimberger suffered from abdominal pains which did not improve with treatment. With the help of one of his colleagues, gallstones were diagnosed. He had to undergo surgery. The weekend before the scheduled date of surgery, Hans Wimberger went on a day trip to the Dachstein mountain massif planning to come back in a week or two. He was a very optimistic man. On Wednesday, October 13, he underwent surgery which was complicated by kidney failure and coma. He died on October 16, 1954. ◆

Bibliography

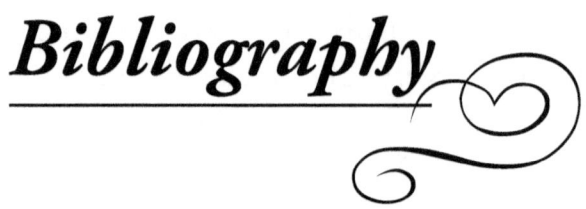

Albers-Schönberg H.
Röntgenbilder einer seltenen Knochenerkrankung.
Münch Med Wochenschr 1904;51:365.

Albers-Schönberg H.
Die Röntgentechnik; Lehrbuch für Ärzte und Studierende.
Hamburg: L. Gräfe & Sillem, 1903.

Baastrup CI.
On the spinous processes of the lumbar vertebrae and the soft tissue
between them, and on pathological changes in that region.
Acta Radiol 1933;14:52-54

Edling L.
Christian Ingerslev Baastrup: in memoriam.
Acta Radiol 1951;35:326-30

Carman RD, Miller A.
The Roentgen Diagnosis of Diseases of the Alimentary Canal.
Philadelphia: Saunders, 1917

Brown LR.
A tribute to Russell Daniel Carman.
Mayo Clin Proc 1995;70:1215-7.

Chilaiditi D.
Zur Frage der Hepatoptose und Ptose im allgemeinen im Anschluss an drei Fälle von temporärer, partieller Leberverlagerung. Fortschr Röntgenstr 1910;16:173-208

Walsh SD, Cruikshank JG.
Chilaiditi syndrome. Age Ageing 1977;6:51-57

Beclere A.
Rectification d'une erreur de diagnostic: ectopie du colon transverse prise a l'examen radioscopique, pour un abces gazeux sousphrenique. Bull Mem Soc Med Hop Paris 1899;16:506-507

Codman EA.
Bone Sarcoma, an Interpretation of the Nomenclature Used by the Committee of the Registry of Bone Sarcoma of the American College of Surgeons. New York: P. B. Hoeber, 1925.

Codman EA.
The Shoulder. Boston: Thomas Todd Co, 1934.

Neuhauser D.
Ernest Amory Codman MD.
Qual Saf Health Care 2002;1:104-105

Doppler C.
Über das farbige Licht der Doppelsterne und einiger anderer Gestirne des Himmels. Abhandlungen der königlichen böhmischen Gesellschaft der Wissenschaften 1843;2:465-482

Doppler C.
Bemerkungen zu meiner Theorie des farbigen Lichtes der Doppelsterne, mit vorzüglicher Rücksicht auf die von Herrn Dr. Ballot in Utrecht dagegen erhobenen Bedenken.
Annalen der Physik 1846;68:1-35

O'Connor JJ, Robertson EF.
MacTutor History of Mathematics.
On: http://www.mcs.st-and.ac.uk/

Roguin A.
Christian Johann Doppler: the man behind the effect.
Br J Radiol 2002;75:615-619

Fleischner F.
Plattenformige Atelektasen in der Unterlappen der Lunge. Fortschr
Röntgenstr 1936;54:315-321

Fleischner F, Hampton AO, Castleman B.
Linear shadows in the lung. AJR 1941;46:610-618

Fleischner F.
Unilateral pulmonary embolism with increased compensatory
circulation through the unoccluded lung.
Radiology 1959;73:591-597.

Fleischner F.
on http://bidmc.harvard.edu/sites/bidmc/home.asp

Fraenkel E.
Untersuchungen über die Möller-Barlowsche Krankheit.
Fortschr Röntgenstr 1903-4;7;231-265, 291-310

Fraenkel E.
Archiv und Atlas der normalen und pathologischen Anatomie in
typischen Röntgenbildern. Hamburg, 1910

Fraenkel E.
Die kongenitale Knochensyphilis im Röntgenbilde. Archiv und
Atlas der normalen und pathologischen Anatomie. Hamburg: Gräfe
& Sillem, 1911

Golden R.
The effect of bronchostenosis upon the roentgen ray shadow in carcinoma of the bronchus. AJR 1925;13:21-30

Rigler LG.
In memoriam. Ross Golden, M.D. 1890-1975.
Radiology 1975;116:742-743.

Hampton AO, Castleman B.
Correlation of postmortem chest teleroentgenograms with autopsy findings. AJR 1940;43:305-326

Hampton AO, Schumacher FV.
Radiographic differentiation of benign and malignant gastric ulcers.
Clin Symp 1956;8:161-171

Schatzki R, Lingley JR.
Aubrey O. Hampton, 1900-1955. AJR 1956;75:396-97

Hounsfield GN.
Autobiography. On: http://nobelprize.org

Engineers and Inventors.
New York: Peter Bedrick Books; 1986:85-86

Di Chiro G, Brooks RA.
The 1979 Nobel Prize in Physiology or Medicine.
Science 1979:1060-1062

Kerley P.
Lung changes in acquired heart disease. AJR 1958;80:256-63

Simpson L.
Irish contributions to our understanding of heart disease.
Heart Lung Circ 2003;12 Suppl 2:73-77

Peter James Kerley.
Lancet 1979 Mar 31;1(8118):735

Peter James Kerley
http://www.authorandbookinfo.com/ngcoba/ke.htm

Naclerio EA.
The V sign in the diagnosis of spontaneous rupture of the esophagus (an early roentgen clue).
Am J Surg 1957;93:291-8

Ackert K.
King on his court. Cardozo coach honors dad & revered patient.
NY Daily News, January 20, 2003

Sinha R.
Naclerio's V sign.
Radiology 2007;245:296-297

Park EA, Guild HI, Jackson D, Bond M.
The recognition of scurvy with especial reference to the early x-ray changes.
Arch Dis Childhood 1935;10: 265-294.

Jackson D, Park EA.
Congenital scurvy. A case report.
J Pediatr 1935;7:741-753.

Edwards A. Park.
Pediatrics 1969;44;897-901

Pelkan KF.
The roentgenogram in early scurvy.
Am J Dis Child 1925; 30: 174-88
San Jose Mercury News, April 24, 1992:78

Rigler LG.
Spontaneous pneumoperitoneum: a roentgenologic sign found in the supine position.
Radiology 1941;37:604-607

Lewicki AM.
The Rigler sign and Leo G. Rigler.
Radiology 2004;233:7-12

Schatzki R, Gary JE.
Dysphagia due to a diaphragm-like localized narrowing in the lower esophagus (lower esophageal ring). AJR 1953;70:911-922.

Schatzki R, Gary JE.
The lower esophageal ring. AJR 1956;75:246-261.

Hebenstreit, Uta.
Die Verfolgung jüdischer Ärzte in Leipzig in den Jahren der nationalsozialistischen Diktatur: Schicksale der Vertriebenen.
Dissertation, 1997, Leipzig, p. 142.

Schatzki SC.
Richard Schatzki, M.D.: a biography. AJR 1988;150:508-509.

Spalding AB.
A pathognomonic sign of intra-uterine death.
Surg Gynecol Obstet 1922; 34: 754

Handler LC.
Overlapping of the fetal skull bones in breech presentation.
SA J Radiology 1964;(March) 21:15-18

McLeary RD.
An early sign of fetal demise.
Radiology 1982;142:712

Thomson JL.
The differential diagnosis of Spalding's sign.
Br J Radiol 1950;23:122-124

Stierlin E.
Die Radiographie in der Diagnostik der Ileozoekaltuberkulose
und anderer Krankheiten des Dickdarms.
Münch Med Wochenschr 1911:58:1231-1235

Stierlin E.
Klinische Röntgendiagnostik des Verdauungskanals. Bearbeitet auf
Grund des Material der chirurgischen Universitätskliniken Basel
und Zürich. Wiesbaden, J.F. Bergmann, 1916

Stierlin E, Vischer A.
Chirurgische Beobachtungen auf allen Etappen im serbisch-
türkischen Kriege 1912—1913. Aus der Chirurgischen Klinik in
Basel (Direktor: Prof. Dr. F. de Quervain).

Sauerbruch F.
Eduard Stierlin. Münch Med Wochenschr 1919;12 December:1445

Frankel VH.
The Terry-Thomas sign. Clin Orthop Relat Res 1977;129:321-322

Thomas T.
Filling the Gap. Toronto; Clarke, Irwin Inc., 1959

Westermark N.
On the roentgen diagnosis of lung embolism: brief review of the
incidence, pathology and clinical symptoms of lung embolism. Acta
Radiol 1938; 357-372

http://en.wikipedia.org/wiki/Nils_Westermark;
last accessed: July 18, 2009

Wimberger, Hans.
Zur Diagnose des Sauglingsskorbuts.
Zeitschrift für Kinderheilkunde 1923; 36: 279

Wimberger H.
Klinisch-radiologische Diagnostik v. Rachitis, Scorbut u. Lues im
Kindesalter. Ergebn. d. inner. Med. u. Kinderheilkunde 1925; 28:
264

Wimberger, Hans.
Der Säuglingsskorbut in Wien 1916–1923.
Europ J Pediatr 1924; 38: 293-300

**Chick H, Dalyell EJ, Hume M, Mackay HMM, Smith HH,
Wimberger Hans.**
Aus der Universitäts-Kinderklinik in Wien. Über die Ätiologie der
Rachitis im Säuglingsalter. Beobachtungen über Prophylaxe und
Heilung.
Europ J Pediatr 1922; 34(1-4): 75-93

**Chick H, Dalyell EJ, Hume M, Mackay MM, Smith HH,
Wimberger H.**
The etiology of rickets in infants. Prophylatic and curative
observations at the Vienna University Kinder Klinik.
Lancet 1922; 2: 7-12.

Chick H, Hume M.
The work of the Accessory Food Factors Committee.
Br Med Bull 1956; 12: 5-8

Photographic Credits

H.E.Albers-Schönberg
Published with permission from National Library of Medicine.

C.I.Baastrup
Reproduced from: Edling L. Christian Ingerslev Baastrup: in memoriam. Acta Radiologica 1951; 35: 326-330. With permission from Informa Healthcare.

R.Carman; Carman meniscus sign
Reproduced from: Kanne J, Rohrmann CA jr, Lichtenstein JE. Eponyms in radiology of the digestive tract: historical perspectives and imaging appearance. Radiographics 2006; 26: 129-142. Published with permission from Dr.J.Kanne and Radiographics.

Swett and Lewis
From http://www.electrotherapymuseum.com

D.Chilaiditi
Courtesy of Gerry Livadas.

E.A.Codman
Published with permission from National Library of Medicine.

Codman triangle
Published with permission from MiASoft Systems Ltd.

F.G.Fleischner
From the inheritance of Guido Holzknecht. Published with permission of the Medical University of Vienna.

Fleischner lines
Published with permission of Dr.K.Karuppasamy.

Fleischner sign
Reproduced from: Marshall GB, Farnquist BA, MacGregor JH, Burrowes PW. Signs in thoracic imaging. J Thorac Imaging 2006; 21: 76-90. Published with permission of Dr.P.Burrowes and Wolters-Kluwer.

E.Fraenkel
Published with permission from National Library of Medicine.

Fraenkel line
Published with permission from MiASoft Systems Ltd.

Ross Golden, Ross Golden and his baseball team
Courtesy of David Kusel.

Golden sign
Reproduced from: Marshall GB, Farnquist BA, MacGregor JH, Burrowes PW. Signs in thoracic imaging. J Thorac Imaging 2006; 21: 76-90. Published with permission of Dr.P.Burrowes and Wolters-Kluwer.

A.O.Hampton
Reproduced from: Schatzki R, Lingley JR. Aubrey O Hampton 1900-1955. AJR 1956; 75: 396-397. Reprinted with permission from the American Journal of Roentgenology.

Hampton line
Published with permission from Dr.W.Herring and LearningRadiology.com

G.N.Hounsfield
Published with permission from National Library of Medicine.

P.J.Kerley
Reproduced from: Simpson L. Irish contributions to our understanding of heart disease. Heart Lung Circ 2003; 12 Suppl 2: S73-S77. Published with permission from Elsevier.

R.Kienböck with junior physicians.
Published with permission of the Medical University of Vienna.

E.A.Naclerio
Courtesy of Ronald Naclerio.

Naclerio V-sign
Reproduced from: Sinha R. Naclerio's V sign. Radiology 2007; 245: 296-297. Published with permission from Dr. R Sinha and Radiology.

E.A.Park
Reproduced from: Taussig HB. Edwards A Park 1878-1969. J Pediatr 1970; 77: 10. Published with permission from Elsevier.

Park's corner
Reproduced from: Park EA, Guild HI, Jackson D, Bond M. The recognition of scurvy with especial reference to the early x-ray changes. Arch Dis Childhood 1935;10:265-94. Published with permission from BMJ Publishing Group Ltd.

K.Pelkan
Courtesy of Jennifer McCaffrey.

List of passengers of *Kronprinzessin Cecilie, Passport application*
Published with permission from ancestry.com

Pelkan spurs
Published with permission from MiASoft Systems Ltd.

L.G.Rigler
Published with permission from National Library of Medicine.

R.Schatzki
Courtesy of Dr.S.C.Schatzki.

SS Bremen
Photograph from German Federal Archive.

List of passengers Bremen
Published with permission from ancestry.com

A.B.Spalding
Courtesy of Robin Spalding.

Spalding sign
Published with permission from Radiopaedia.org

Stierlin sign
Reproduced from: Pereira JM, Madureira AJ, Vieira A, Ramos I. Abdominal tuberculosis: imaging. Europ J Radiology 2005;55:173-180. Published with permission of Dr. Pereira JM and Elsevier.

N.J.H.Westermark
Published with permission of Dr.Torbjörn Andersson, Stockholm.

Westermark sign
Reproduced from: Westermark N. On the Roentgen diagnosis of lung embolism. Acta Radiologica 1938; 19: 357-372. Published with permission from Informa Healthcare.

H.Wimberger
Courtesy of Gerhard Wimberger.

Wimberger sign
Courtesy of Dr.Lakshmana Das Narla, Richmond, VA

Wimberger ring
Published with permission from MiASoft Systems Ltd.

About the author

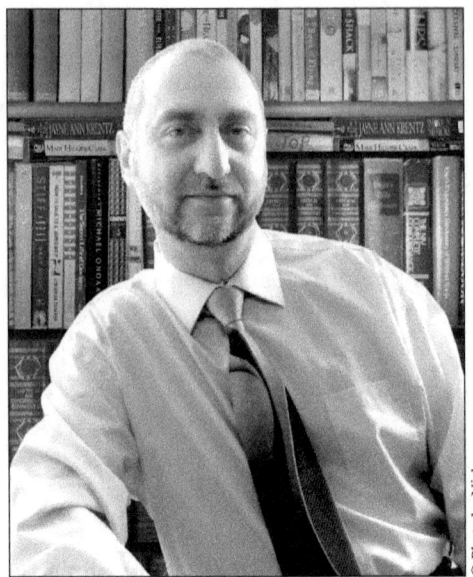

© Photo by Nick

Years ago, at the age of five, he was taken by his father, Dr. Samuel N. Maizlin, a talented surgeon and an outstanding military officer, to the history museum and on a walk through the fields of almost forgotten wars. Since that time, Zeev Maizlin has had careers in surgery and the military before landing in radiology. Now he is a staff radiologist, Associate Professor of Radiology, and an author of more than twenty works. Apparently, that early historical touch prevailed in his further studies and training and developed into a life-long interest in history. This led to a confidence that the past is connected to the present and its knowledge is essential for the future. Convinced that the professional interests are not to be limited to everyday routine, inspired and supported by his family and friends, he tries to unveil secrets and mysteries of the past and to evoke curiosity in his colleagues and trainees.

Further books in this series:

- *Mysteries behind invention of CT scanner.*

- *Ancient myths and modern radiology.*

- *Divine proportion and radiology.*

- *Fatal weapons and radiology.*